HEALED BY FARM

And Why Americans Die Too Young

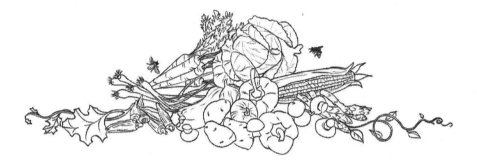

"THE GREATEST LIFE-SAVING BOOK EVER WRITTEN"

JOHN RANKIN

This book is intended as a healthy eating and lifestyle reference guide only and not as a medical manual. The information provided herein is shared to help you make informed decisions about your health. It is not intended as a substitute for any treatment that may have been prescribed by your doctor. If you suspect that you have a medical problem, we urge you to seek competent medical help.

Mention of specific companies, organizations, or authorities in this book does not imply endorsement by the author or publisher, nor does mention of specific companies, organizations, or authorities imply that they endorse this book, it's author, or the publisher.

ISBN: 978-1-7322562-0-0

Cover Designer: Bradley Clark

Editor: Judy Hansen

TABLE OF CONTENTS

FORWARD

I first met John Rankin just a couple of months after the cardiac event that by all rights should have killed him. I'm the manager of the supplement and body care department of a popular health food supermarket, and he was looking for a good fish oil. He was also still furious that he'd woken up with a stent and prescriptions for statin drugs and blood thinners, and was absolutely determined that that situation was going to be as short-termed as possible. In the first five minutes of our conversation, I learned that he already knew a great deal about wellness and nutrition, and was adding to his knowledge at warp speed---and I also knew that he could out-talk anybody I'd ever met.

Over the past few years, John has become a good friend of mine----and anyone else who'll listen. I trust his advice because I've seen it work, and know how much time he spends researching the latest information available.

Taking control of your health isn't always easy (I'm living proof of that), but his advice has made a huge difference in the health of my own family and many others. On the fourth day after cutting sugar out of my diet, my chronically inflamed joints just unlocked, and I felt years younger. I'm trying hard not to backslide, and I'm lucky to have him around as my own Jiminy Cricket (conscience), pushing me to do better.

I've watched John coach other people, and the results have

been extraordinary. I've also seen how sad he is when some of those people who've done so well start sliding back into those old bad habits. It's not a matter of ego for John, but it is personal----he really does want everyone to live a long and healthy life.

Do yourself a favor: listen to what he has to say, then clean up your act.

Be strong, follow John Rankin's way, and live well to a very old age!

– Kathy Goodbuddy

INTRODUCTION
"Blood tests don't lie."

Greetings and welcome to the John Rankin Way. "Healed By Farm" is the story of how this "Way" was created, and it will be the last health care book you'll ever need. For starters I'd like to suggest that before you read even a single paragraph of this book, stop and ask yourself why you are attracted to a self-healing book. Are you or a loved-one suffering from a sickness or even a horrific disease? Is someone close to you dying or even just overweight, desperately needing help but unable to find it? Are you frustrated that you or your loved-ones have been in the care of and following the advice of your so-called health care professional, but instead of getting better you keep getting sicker? I'm guessing you who read this book have many such unanswered questions that keep you seeking. I want you to know that if up to now you haven't found all of the right help, don't despair. I am here to teach you the answers you are seeking. As I share these precious truths, your life will change for the better....forever.

I've learned how to have consistently and permanently fabulous health, and I am here to share what I've learned. In this book and on my website (*www.johnrankinswayback.com*) you will learn some very special words of wisdom that will change everything about how you look at food and healing the human body. I will teach you how to make today the beginning of the healthiest and best days of your life. I will teach you the things that I personally did that saved my life and made living it fabulous.

In the summer of 2013 when I was just seconds away from meeting my Maker, the direction of my life changed forever and I will never look back. From being at death's door to becoming an extremely strong and healthy person--with the vitality and blood test levels of a teenager--my path is one you can't refuse to consider. I'm here to challenge you folks, to awaken you out of your complacency and confusion. If you will read and learn and make the same wise choices I did, in just a few short months your health and your life will dramatically improve.

I learned for myself that blood tests don't lie. I used my ever-improving test results to document how to heal my own body. I call these truths the elixir of life. It is my belief that as long as I keep doing what I have learned, I will never be sick again. I may even fitfully fly right past my goal of living to be one hundred years old! I don't doubt that (God-willing) this is very possible. I will teach you how to improve your blood tests to reach peak health. Being in the range on blood tests is not something to be proud of. Being on the edge of that range is not the kind of healthy I'm talking about either. I want you to become and live on the absolute top of your game.

I learned these truths the hard way, and I know what I'm talking about. I have connected a lot of dots to make sense of what works and why. I have done the work for you. I have learned the truth our ancestors knew, and I am bringing it back. Listen and learn, folks. This is all you need to know to keep yourself out of the doctor's office and out of the hospital beds. It's not rocket science. It's simple, common sense truth about food.

Maybe you think you have been spared poor health, but none of you in this western civilization will escape the grim reaper if you keep eating what is culturally popular. All of you are becoming addicted to the very things that destroy health, and you don't even know it. By becoming addicted, your freedom to be healthy is being stolen from you unaware. You are giving away your power blindly. You are most likely eating fake food that even in small amounts is poisoning your body and blocking it's natural ability to heal itself.

I'm guessing most of you are on some kind of prescription medication or combination of such. You may think by doing so that your body is getting better with those prescriptions. But you are being slowly put to sleep. You happily go along thinking you have your meds and you get along just fine. You think this is normal, but normal because of drugs is absolutely not normal. Wouldn't you like to get so healthy that you never have to think of taking a drug again?

But you may say that you like your eating habits and you don't intend to become disciplined about food. To that I say, "go ahead on that path and almost die like I did--or even worse." But if you have even a little wisdom floating around in that head of yours, you will get your wake-up call vicariously with my story and save yourself and your loved-ones a lot of hell. You are being dumbed down by the medical world to believe the food in America is approved by the FDA so it must be just fine. It is not just fine--it is anything but. Wake up America! Get a handle on this before it is too late. You can reverse any disease--starting right now. This is a God-given mission I'm on, and like Jonah in the Bible story, I can't avoid it. I'm sharing the truth, and you can take it or leave it.

God bless America--we surely need it. The process of dumbing down Americans to buy and eat products in the name of food is alive and well, poisoning the bodies of innocent victims for profit. By explaining the difference with our modern-day eating habits and the way our ancestors ate, I explain the bigger picture. I sincerely hope it helps you to wake up and take charge of your health. It is my heart's desire that we join forces to drain the swamp of fake food in America.

Today's news describes the horrific stories of babies born to drug and alcohol-addicted mothers. We have heard it almost daily and are deeply saddened yet perhaps don't identify because it hasn't happened to our family or friends. The stories are heartbreaking and we are so happy to think we were spared. But were we really spared? I was born in December of 1956 as an innocent victim myself, soon to become addicted to a poison far worse than alcohol--in a way no one would have known. This is how my story began.

There is no one to blame. My good parents were only con-forming to the advice given to them by the doctor (backed by scientists, the US Agriculture Department and the industrial-ized American food industry). Well it's a good thing we have the government and the food companies looking out for our health, right?

This book tells the story of what I have learned--as I said the hard way--through a lifelong process of dealing with death in my family, adding to that much study, prayer, observation, and then that life-changing very personal near-death experience. I hope to answer many questions you might have about the health of your family, friends, loved ones and our nation. I'm not a certified dietician or medical practitioner of any kind nor do I claim to be. But hopefully by the time I get through sharing the real truth about health and how to heal our bodies with real whole foods, you won't have an interest in hearing what certified dietitians have to say anyway. And for the record I don't blame them. They just happen to have drunk the same kool-aid as the rest of the medical profession. I'll explain why I believe this further on. My guess is they haven't done much good for your health either or you wouldn't be reading this book.

Some folks call me fanatical. Some call me extreme. And some call me passionate and inspiring, even a Moses for our day. I see myself as being extremely passionate about learning the truth, especially when it comes to saving lives--starting with my own--using the God-given and universally ordained healing power of real foods that God through Mother Nature intended!

I sincerely hope and pray that the stories and information I share with you in this book will allow you to understand the truth for yourself. As I see it from my perspective now--hindsight--the incredibly true, sad, funny, passionate and very adventurous story of my life was designed exactly for this mission: to find the truth about healing my own body from disease, and to teach with all the passion in my soul how you too can live a healthy and happy life--and inspire your loved-ones to do the same.

HEALED BY FARM
CHAPTER ONE

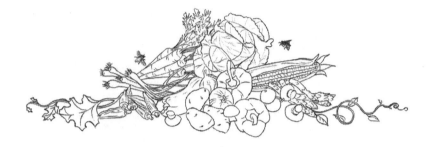

INSTANT ADDICTION

*"The American-food-con has been
alive and well for most of our lifetimes."*

The slow poisoning and addiction to my body started when I was very young. On February 6, 1957, when I was only a six-week old baby, the family doctor gave my mother a prescribed list of things to feed me. The prescription included such suggestions as fruit juices, canned fruit, and if that wasn't already a lot of sugar for a newborn, add this: a handwritten instruction

DR. JACK CHESNEY
~~DR. ROBERT F. YOUNG~~   Dr.R.B. Willingham
129 SHELBOURNE TOWERS APARTMENTS
850-860 SOUTH 20th STREET
KNOXVILLE, TENNESSEE

Date: February 6, 1957

For Baby: John Rankin

Weight: 12 pounds 2½ ounces

Length: 23 5/8" inches

For feeding prepare the following:

Give 2 to 3 ounces of boiled water between feedings.

At 8:00 A.M. or 4:00 P.M., or at other convenient time, give 3 to 4 ounces of undiluted orange, grapefruit, tomato, or pineapple juices. Alternate juice from time to time.

At 8:00 A.M. give   ~~drops of~~

At 10:00 A.M. give 2 to 3 tablespoonsful of Pablum, Clapp Cereal, Cream of Wheat, Gerber Cereal, Wheatena, Oatmeal, or other cooked cereal.

Begin egg yolk – raw, soft poached, or soft boiled. Start with a taste and increase gradually until a whole yolk is given. Do not give egg white until baby is a year old.

Hard boiled egg, well mashed, may later be used. Watch carefully for swollen lips, face rash, vomiting, or other evidence of sensitivity to egg.

At 2:00 P.M. give ¼ can of canned baby vegetables or vegetable soup or 3 tablespoonsful of home pureed vegetables or soup. Simple vegetable mixtures may be given.

At 6:00 P.M. begin pureed fruit such as apple sauce, prunes, pears, peaches, or mixtures. These may be canned baby fruit or may be pureed at home. Begin with a teaspoonful and increase gradually to 2 or 3 tablespoonsful. Later offer small amount of ripe banana.

Also give baby cereal as at 10:00 A.M.

list on how to mix bottles of 'sugarized' formula for me.

"Mix 13 to 16 ounces of evaporated milk with 16 ounces of boiled water and 3 tablespoons of corn syrup."

Corn syrup is a concentrated solution of refined processed glucose and other sugars derived from cornstarch. The original versions of dark corn syrup had significant amounts of a sugar alcohol called sorbitol. Doctors at the time of my birth were recommending (under the influence of the refined food industry) bottle feeding instead of breastfeeding, prescribing these homemade formulas that included corn syrup meant to ward off constipation in the babies. I have learned to my surprise this same prescription for constipation is still given today.

Scientific studies prove that corn syrup actually causes diarrhea, bloating, nausea and vomiting in infants. Well there you go! If giving your newborn baby processed refined foods made from cornstarch and loaded with sugar alcohols is not enough to scare you, then maybe intentionally hurting your baby's stomach or making them vomit is. Did you ever wonder why your baby got constipated in the first place? Just like an adult, they are given foods that are full of processed refined sugars and cornstarch--not real food.

Ever since my wife and I had our first child, I have heard people say things such as, 'You shouldn't get in the sun when you're pregnant,' or 'You should eat this or take that or breathe this way or sleep in a certain way.' So yes, I believe people are always seeking to do what is best. I have overheard conversations or read studies that will suggest that the baby should eat certain foods or not eat certain foods. Isn't it a sad day when babies can't even poop without giving them drugs or calling the doctor to ask what to feed them? What has happened to our society and mostly good ole-fashioned common sense like breast-feeding or unprocessed, unrefined REAL FOOD?

A word of warning for new expectant mothers: between your best friend, doctor, cousin, sister, or a well-followed website, someone is going to try to convince you that breast milk is just not as good as formula and that your new baby can't survive without the special mix of the all new refined healthy 96-ingredient vitamin infused Turbo 2000 drink. (GIVE ME A BREAK!!)

How have babies survived all of these years without these perfect new improved formulas? Well that's just my point: proof is the state of health in America since the industrialized food industry. They have created dozens of new and improved foods that are supposedly the only thing that's going to save your baby. They have even taught this propaganda in second and third-world countries, opposing the norm of breastfeeding, scaring mothers into doubting their own nature. Well folks, this is what is called greedy untruthful marketing.

The big companies making processed refined (fake) foods have only one goal: to improve profits for their shareholders by selling you whatever they can get you addicted to, and taking your money for it. I don't believe they care about you, your family, or your health. They constantly bombard us through false marketing practices and quote scientific studies that are done by none other than their own paid employees. If you think you are immune to these con's, just look at your children's bubble gum (sugar) flavored toothpaste that (yours truly) bought them. As you read on in this book you will learn much more of the truth about 'fake food.'

As you can see from classic ads from over fifty years ago, these non-accountable marketing schemes are not new. The American-food-con has been alive and well for most of our lifetimes.

Breast milk is unequaled in nutrition for babies. There is no milk substitute on this planet that can replicate the immune

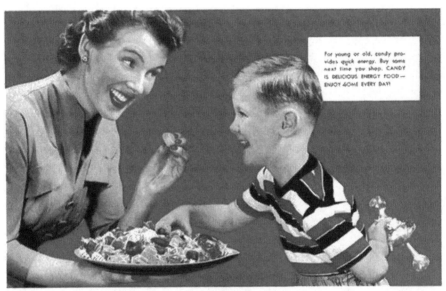

For young or old, candy provides quick energy. Buy some next time you shop. CANDY IS DELICIOUS ENERGY FOOD — ENJOY SOME EVERY DAY!

Kids <u>need</u> the energy candy gives

HERE'S WHY SMART MOTHERS BUY CANDY IN CELLOPHANE

properties that a mother passes on to her child through breast milk. Regardless of what the label says, the sugared-up inflammatory modern formulated milk powders can never replicate the natural fat, carbohydrates, and proteins that are found in a mother's breast milk. I understand there are exceptions when mothers cannot nurse for health reasons and have to do the best they can, but for most of the mothers in this world, that is not an issue.

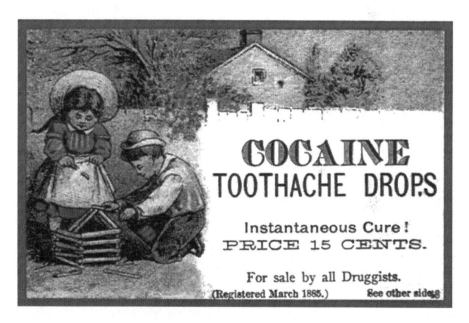

The true fact is that a baby needs its mother's natural milk for brain development and body growth. The good health of a baby's body is created by its mother's gut bacteria, and every living cell, organ, muscle, and bone in a newborn child is the result of what a mother eats. When an expectant mother drinks sugary insulin-damaging drinks, eats hydrogenated fast-food trans fat, and consumes prescription medications daily, then would you expect her potentially marvelous beautiful baby to

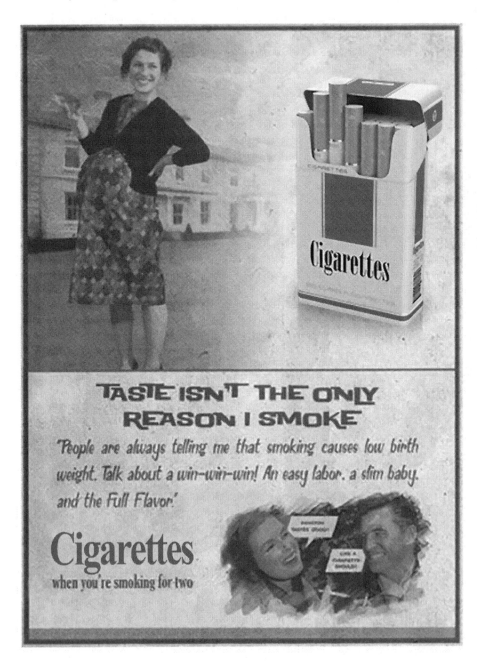

Start 'Em Out Young!

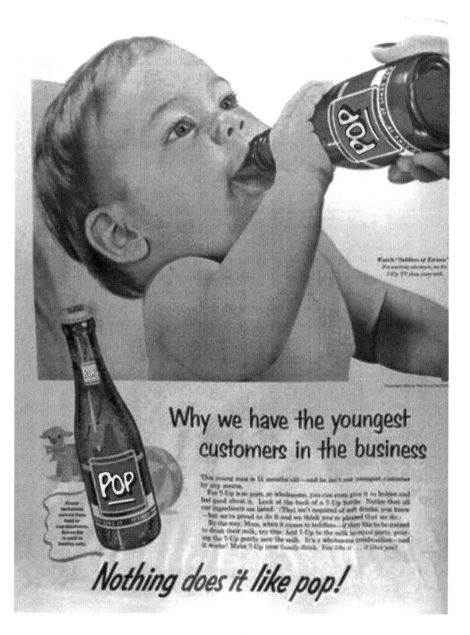

be anything but sick? On the flipside if an expectant mother consumes foods like healthy organic fruits, vegetables, seeds, nuts, eggs from grass-fed chickens, plus poultry, beef, and raw dairy, then the result will be quite different with awesome, healthy, beautiful babies coming into this world--without so many bad health issues.

The small intestine is approximately 85% of the human immune system. The old saying, 'You are what you eat" has become absolutely true. Through some of the latest scientific studies we learn that good gut bacteria is the answer to good health, and for good reason. I believe it's the secret to life. If an expectant mother eats nothing but 'fake food', then her gut flora will be ruined. It is the result of the mother's good gut bacteria that feeds the fetus while in the womb. Knowing this fact, it shouldn't be a news flash that babies are born into this world with things like attention deficit disorder, bipolarism, autism and cancer. And yes, the latest studies are actually proving a correlation between good and bad gut bacteria as being the cause of these illnesses.

As an example, if you water and feed your garden with clean spring water and natural organic fertilizers, it will evolve into something wonderful that mother nature intended for us to ingest to stay healthy. The produce of such a garden will actually create beautiful gut flora that builds your immune system to perfection. If you feed your garden with polluted water and chemical fertilizers that are out of balance with nature, then such produce will do the opposite to your gut, even killing your good bacteria which will in effect lower your immune system to very dangerous unhealthy levels.

It is definitely a mother's responsibility to keep herself healthy during and after pregnancy. I have seen many mothers eat a very healthy diet during pregnancy, only to celebrate after nine long months by going back after delivery to their old food and drinking habits. The truth is that while you nurse your baby with milk from your body, the foods you eat should be solely 100% from Mother Nature's bounties. And just so you know, manufactured baby formulas today are made of approximately 55% highly addictive disease-causing inflammatory refined sugars, not to mention the MSG and other dangerous chemicals hidden in the labeling.

Fathers, don't think you are off the hook and without responsibility. A father not only plays a huge role at the time of conception, but also in the way he leads his wife and children and the example he sets for them. The overall health of children can be determined by whether the father is healthy or unhealthy, whether he is an alcoholic or sugarholic, lazy or athletic. A wise word to fathers is to constantly help your wife and family search for all-natural healthy foods. The reward for your discipline? You will have smarter, healthier, calmer, and more obedient children. You will save tens of thousands of dollars in healthcare. And you will enjoy a beautiful relationship with a wife who lives free of chemically-induced, hormone-driven anxiety after giving childbirth.

I do understand a father's concern for paying for the more expensive all-natural healthy food and breaking the family grocery budget. But when you feed your body solely with grass-fed meats, fish, raw dairy, nuts, seeds, organic fruits and vegetables all day long, then your liver will no longer crave the junk food that you spend so much of your money on. Just cutting out one junk-food item per day (such as soda) for you and your spouse at a fast-food restaurant on weekdays only will save you upwards of seventy dollars per month. Small changes such as this can make it possible for you and your family to enjoy all of the wonderful health benefits you desire. And as an added bonus: you will be able to really taste the beautiful flavors of real food that can only be discerned when refined processed sugars are eliminated from your diet.

So make your choice, folks: enjoy all the goodness of life Mother Nature intended in keeping us healthy from birth, or continue to be addicted to sugars and believe the deceptive marketing schemes of the conspiring refined-food industry that unfortunately has been taking your money selling you 'fake food' from the first day we entered this world and through all the years since.

HEALED BY FARM
CHAPTER TWO

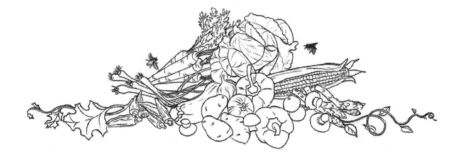

CLIMBING THE CABINETS

"A sugar-addicted child will steal, beg and borrow to get their sugar high. What are your kids doing when not in your protective care?"

When I was two or three years old, I quickly became consciously aware of what my taste buds liked the most, and I can assure you it wasn't brussel sprouts! My mother was a great cook, and living in a family of seven (I was the youngest) meant that we had seven birthday cakes per year plus all of the traditional holiday cookies, cakes, and candy. I learned at a very young age that I loved these treats made with processed sugar, at least my brain told me so. It's very sad that my brain didn't also tell me about the very real consequences of eating sugar and what a high price my body would have to pay for the next fifty-three years. Little did I know that I was setting myself up for a health disaster and was already highly addicted to refined sugars from birth.

It was also unfortunate that I became aware at three years old that I didn't have to wait any longer for holidays or birthdays to get my sugar (drug) fix. My father had taught me to fall in love with his jelly beans and all kinds of assorted store bought highly addictive candies. He would occasionally bring these treasures out of hiding and share a few with me. I was already addicted to refined processed sugars from my baby formula, and being that little 'information kid' that I was only meant that I just had to know more about these treats! My father would magically make these delicious treasures appear (or at least it seemed that way). He always had them, but I was certain we didn't have anything like that in our house since I never saw him put them away. I remember looking in every drawer in the house that I could reach trying to discover his hiding place--only to find nothing.

Then one day when my father had his candy out, my little brain went to work and I followed him, watching to discover where he put them away. And I was delighted to discover where they were: in a small cabinet way up high over our refrigerator! (Always remember: your kids are watching)! And then something happened inside me. It was like showing the cat where the mouse is. At last I knew where to get my sugar (drug) fix without even having to ask anyone!

The problem was a few things were in my way. Number one was that if my father caught me sneaking into something I wasn't supposed to be in, there would have been a hanging before the trial. Secondly, living in a household of five children meant someone was always roaming around the house, and if my siblings caught me they would certainly turn me into the authorities. And lastly came the problem of getting to the cabinet above the refrigerator at barely four years old. The cabinet was so high up it might as well have been Mount Everest. I had to put a plan into action!

Was it worth it for me to risk sudden death by my father, get turned in by my siblings (or worse--beat up and then turned in)? And then there was just one last big hurdle: how to climb up there without killing myself. What a sad tale: if I had only known the very thing I was climbing for was actually the thing that was going to try to take my life decades later.

So there I was facing this huge dilemma and putting together my strategy as if it were a military war plan. I came to the conclusion that the best time to put my plan into action was when my father was at work and my siblings were scattered around the house--or better yet the neighborhood. I wasn't worried as much about my mother. Remember, I was the baby!

I thought about this for a few days and then realized I would have to push a chair twenty feet across the kitchen and climb the chair to the countertop--just to find out that I was only halfway there to my drug fix. Although my father's candy was in the cabinet above the refrigerator, there I stood on the countertop looking up (and waiting for the search lights to come on with rifles firing any moment). Then I started climbing between the refrigerator and the wall in a one-foot gap, squeezing upward until my small skinny little body was sitting on top of the refrigerator!

I remember sitting there looking downward at the floor and wondering just what have I done now and what kind of trouble was I facing if caught. Apparently my addiction was more important as I turned and opened the small cabinet door and there it was--the golden prize that my brain had determined was the only thing that would give me joy and happiness: a bag of jellybeans, and certainly not just any bag. At that moment it was my bag. Well, it felt that way, but I only took enough that my father would not miss them. I remember that day sitting high up in the air chewing on the sugar and thinking I was in heaven. Thinking back to that time now, I shudder, knowing the horrific health effects this sugar was actually creating--the consequences being quite the opposite of heaven.

Over the next couple of years before I entered school, I became even more highly addicted to refined processed sugars and foods. I had unlimited access to candy via the top cabinet that I had conquered (and eventually mastered my climbing skills on). My family no longer owns that house, but I would love to go back there and look for my claw marks left in the knotty pine wall beside the refrigerator.

Little did I or my parents realize what was happening to me or what kind of future I was setting myself up for (maybe like your kids). I was so extremely sugared-up as a child that, unfortunately, I was accused of everything from being attention-deficit to being maybe just a little crazy to even being a very bad boy--none of which of course was true. A sugar-addicted child will steal, beg and borrow to get their sugar high. What are your kids doing when not in your protective care?

HEALED BY FARM

CHAPTER THREE

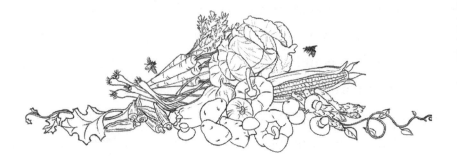

LEAVING HOME FOR SCHOOL

"Instead of being a normal little five-year old first grade boy like most children, I was a drug (sugar) addicted dealer."

It was the big day I could hardly wait for. No, not college--first grade at Sterchi Elementary School. Even at the young age of five, I was not the least bit afraid to climb onto the big yellow school bus and enter a school with older kids. I had two older brothers and two older sisters who would surely protect me from anything, at least that's what I thought! But there was one thing they couldn't protect me from: my addiction to sugar and refined processed foods.

By that early time in my life, I was as addicted to sugar as a drug addict was to heroin. Consequently, those dangerous free radicals were already eating away my body like maggots eating a piece of meat, due to the total inflammation of every cell in my body from eating so much sugar.

I was in school less than a few days when I discovered something magical: a small store that sold goodies. My wildest dreams just became a reality--a store inside of the school. The store was usually operated by a couple of well-behaved kids. Needless to say, I was never chosen to work there for the thirty minutes it was open each day prior to school starting.

I quickly learned the store had some really cool things like notebook paper, pencils, rulers, big gummy erasers, and cherry cough drops. Yep, cherry cough drops. And once I tasted them I immediately realized I was about to have the next dilemma in my life. I vividly remember patiently waiting in line to buy my first box of the delicious red sugar drops. I wondered if they would even sell a first grader--someone as young as I--something that was considered cough medicine.

As the line shortened, I remember nervously thinking that I might be facing a trip to the principal's office just for asking for them (when it was obvious I did not even have a cough). But thankfully I didn't end up in kiddie jail that day making what I thought was an illegal purchase.

As I entered Mrs. Payton's first grade class and took my seat, I immediately realized I had another hurdle to jump through. As my mouth watered just thinking about what was in my pocket, I had to figure out just how to open the loud plastic wrapper, then the box, and finally the wax paper packet inside the box--all without getting caught by Mrs. Payton!

Well let me tell you folks, no one can do a three-step candy box opening one handed inside your pocket while pretending to read and write with the other hand better than I can. I slipped them out and into my mouth at the rate of about one every fifteen minutes--and then it became every ten minutes--and then every five.

It wasn't very long until I realized that my classmates didn't have or couldn't afford any cough drops, after all they were five cents per box! Oh yes, five cents was big money in those days, and most students only came to school with their lunch boxes or a quarter to buy a school cafeteria lunch. I on the other hand had parents who were very industrious, making jobs available to my siblings and I which allowed us to earn money from a very young age. I had my own hard-earned money available for at least one box of candy cough drops per day.

My next dilemma was that before long my sugar addiction grew to two, three, even four boxes during each school day. I quickly had to come up with a plan to pay for this new form of feeding my addiction. Bright boy that I was, I soon realized that my first-grade buddies also cherished the flavor of cherry sugar, and the only difference between them and me was that they could not afford the five cent price tag to buy them! And again being the wise little budding entrepreneur I was and the fact that my fifteen to twenty cents per day addiction was breaking me--get where I'm going? Since I very much cherished my twenty-five cents for lunch money that my mom gave me each day, and not being able to use any of that money for my addiction, I of course devised a new plan.

The plan I'm about to tell you about worked brilliantly except for one thing to which I was clueless: it hurt and weakened many of the people who were my close friends, but that was not anywhere in my mind back then. Every single school day, I would buy five or six boxes of the little red drug (sugar) drops. I would then sell my classmates one cough drop at a time for a penny or two until I had recaptured my investment (and had enough left over for myself).

Okay folks, are you starting to see the picture of where this is going? Instead of being a normal little five-year old first grade boy like most children, I was a drug (sugar) addicted dealer. Now parents, just picture your innocent little five-year-old first-grader stepping off the school bus every afternoon with this horrific problem and you never even have the first clue. At such an early age, I was a master at hiding my terrible addiction to sugar--after all, it was an addiction--and I wasn't about to give it up. Your child may not either.

My summer vacation between the first and second grade wasn't as terrible as I feared without my cherry sugar drops. I was finally at the age when I could venture outside of my neighborhood on my bicycle, with the guidance of one or more of my 4 older siblings, of course. And just how long do you think I obeyed those rules set by my parents? After all, I was now a six-year-old addicted drug (sugar) dealer! From this newly learned freedom on my banana seat Schwinn bicycle, I discovered something new only a mile away from home. This place was not only new and exciting, but glorious--a place called Bud's Bicycle Shop.

This place was sent from heaven: new bikes, tires, tubes and a nice old guy named Bud who taught me a lot about how to fix bicycles by myself. Yes, I would just watch him fix bikes while staring right through his big old-fashioned wooden and glass candy case! A summer vacation in Paris couldn't have been better. I now had wheels, spending money, and a road map to candy-ville!

You must understand that Knoxville, Tennessee in 1963 had no big box stores, no chain restaurants, no highway interstate systems, and no poison centers. Yes that's what I now call convenience stores--because other than the occasional small basket of fruit, 99.9% of the ingredients in those stores is basically processed refined sugary products (along with plenty of beer and cigarettes, of course). In those years of my youth, the most common places to buy candy were small mom-and-pop country stores. And at only six years old I had an unforgettable roadmap in my head of at least three of these glorious sugar outlets where I could freely feed my addiction without permission from my parents.

By now most of you must be wondering where in the heck my parents were! Actually I had very responsible loving parents who cared dearly about me and my siblings and taught us about the dangers of life as much as any parent could, with information available at that time. There were just a couple of problems though, one being that in 1963 no one knew the terrible dangers of refined processed sugars and foods (except perhaps politicians and food companies). Sadly and unfortunately most people still don't understand it today. Fortunately for me I do understand the dangers, but had to learn it the hard way. Next, with my parents running their own business, they didn't exactly show up at home with the rest of the rush-hour traffic every day. This equated to my unsupervised daily trip to candyville. Yes, that's exactly what I said, unsupervised. All of that big brother and big sister supervision went right out the door when my oldest brother at age twelve was supposed to be babysitting the younger kids.

How funny looking back--that was like leaving the prisoners with the jail key. My two brothers would often venture a couple of miles from home to a friend's house, and of course they didn't want little brother tagging along. When they saw me trying to follow, they would quickly speed away on their bicycles thinking surely they would lose me. I'm fairly certain my lifelong need for speed may have started at that point when I would often outrun my two sisters--who were also charged with babysitting me--and pursue my brothers on my bicycle. Being the incredibly talented kid that I was (and having the knowledge by eavesdropping of just where their final destination was), I would pedal as fast as I could to join them.

Here is something else to consider with this story: in those days neighborhoods were full of big bad unchained dogs, and at six years old they each seemed like a pack of wolves when they came running from their yards to chase me. Then there were the kids a few streets away in an older neighborhood--referred to as the bad kids. If they saw me riding past their house on my bicycle they would throw rocks, chase me, or even threaten to steal my bicycle and beat me up.

You might wonder why risking my life with such sudden death was so important to me. Oh, I forgot to mention that quite often my adventuresome travels took me right past my new best friend--Bud--and his bicycle/candy shop. And after choosing a square cinnamon sucker, some double bubble gum, a few colored sugar-stuffed straws, and a monster soda,

I eventually arrived at my brother's friend's house and was in their protective custody at last. Needless to say the ride home was quite a bit safer with my bodyguards!

Because of my early start to a horrific addiction, almost daily I would risk being eaten by 'wolves' and 'killed' by the bad kids. Most folks who have ever known me are aware that I can make a bicycle do things it was not built to do. I honestly believe that it all started with those risky sugar-addicted outings! Another way to feed my addiction that I quickly learned from my new freedom (via bicycles) was that every soda bottle lying in a ditch along the roadways had a three-cent return policy from grocery stores. Now picture this: a small child dodging cars while pulling into a grocery store parking lot (daily) riding a banana seat Schwinn one-handed while clutching an extra large bag of bottles with the other. And that two-mile radius of my home had the cleanest ditches in town.

HEALED BY FARM
CHAPTER FOUR

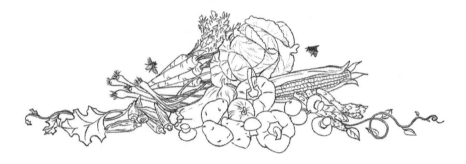

VACATION TO HEAVEN

*"I could hardly wait until my parents
pulled the car into the next cactus-selling,
rattlesnake-viewing, candy-selling gas station."*

My childhood included regular wonderful vacations to heaven--sugar heaven that is, and nobody warned me. Those heavenly vacations were family trips to Arizona to visit my mom's family. Back in those days traveling on busy two-lane highways with a family of seven in a hot non-air-conditioned station wagon was probably not the ideal way to travel, but that was how we rolled back then. It was probably only the five kids who were having any fun, then approximately one-hundred miles from home my father would literally slide the car into a Stuckey's parking lot and scream at all of us to get out of the car.

No, he wasn't really mad at us, just frustrated about the fact that we had totally worn him out in only one-hundred miles, and with seventeen-hundred more to go! Mother would patiently guide all of us through the bathrooms and on to the toys, souvenirs, candy, ice cream, and let's not forget the famous Stuckey's divinity pecan log. Oh yes, everyone over forty-years old has had at least one pecan log in their lifetime.

After herding everyone back into the station wagon and rolling back onto curvy and rolling Highway 70, everything was just great again as my father's foot got heavier on the gas pedal with every mile we passed. Life was grand as we traveled along at warp speed with seven open soda bottles, seven ham and cheese sandwiches with extra mayonnaise, plenty of monster suckers and taffy, and of course the famous pecan roll. Then about one-hundred miles more down the road we stopped again. And no it wasn't because we were hungry. We stopped to clean the trash out of the car! (And of course we had cleaned the car before we left home). It just didn't have stomach increments in the floor when we left our house!

I'm here to testify to you that a hot un-air-conditioned station wagon traveling along at ninety-five miles per hour on curvy hilly two-lane highways with greasy cheesy sugary ingredients in the stomachs of five little kids is a recipe for disaster! Although we repeated these vacation stops year after year without learning our lessons, now as an adult I realize my parents would have stopped anywhere for just a few minutes of silence. I'm very sure they were clueless to the inflammatory responses in their children's bodies from the effects of eating refined processed foods and sugars--no idea at all.

Those early 'modern' days in America seemed like such a wonderful time in history. You could just pull into a restaurant and order some ham sandwiches to go without the owners actually having to first butcher a hog behind the store as in years past. Life was grand as foods were starting to become prepackaged and ready to grab on the run. Potato chips were hitting the shelves with five or six different flavors and kinds to choose from, and some brands even delivered big tasty tins full to your home!

I recently stood in the potato chip aisle--yes I said aisle and not shelf--at my local grocery store and counted 297 different flavors of chips. Every bag on the shelf was made from oxidized, inflammatory, heart-clogging oils, monosodium glutamate, trans fats, refined processed sugars, refined sodium, starches, dyes, fillers, thickeners and "fortified" with synthetic vitamin infusions. The varieties available and the list of dangerous ingredients seemed to never end.

Even though I'm not a fan of white potatoes, they have gotten a bad name lately. Almost all of the chips that I looked at didn't even have any potato in it to start with--just GMO corn, chemicals, and gooey things that studies have proven will kill healthy cells in human beings, especially small children. Through thousands of scientific studies, it has without a doubt been proven that these ingredients will cause everything from cancer to heart disease, diabetes, and Alzheimer's. I surely would have thrown that pecan roll right out the window had I known that, right? No, not really, because remember that by this time in my young life I had already become extremely addicted to sugar and was a thriving cherry cough drop drug dealer as well. Such a choice to give up any candy by an addicted child would have been equivalent to asking a veteran cigarette smoker to throw his favorite pack out the window.

All during that four-day long drive to our vacations in Arizona, I could hardly wait to get to the next state--and it wasn't for the scenery. Don't get me wrong, the western states we traveled through were absolutely gorgeous. But as odd as it may sound I was more concerned with the different flavors of food, soft drinks, and candy which those various states had available. Yes folks, as sad as it sounds, I could hardly wait until my parents pulled the car into the next cactus-selling, rattlesnake-viewing, candy-selling gas station.

Wouldn't it be so very sad if you even thought your young child looked forward to their next vacation stop like a heroin addict looks forward to their next fix? That's exactly what was happening to my small body and what may be happening to yours and one or more of your children's bodies as well. Did I mention that current scientific studies using mice as lab animals have proven that refined processed white sugar is eight times more addictive than cocaine? Think about that the next time you watch Grandma load your children up with soft drinks, donuts, and candy and then say the words, "Oh a little sugar won't hurt them." Grandparents have lots of hard-earned wisdom to share, but the effects of sugar-poisoning is one thing most are clueless about. This is where a parent needs to step up to the plate and make the rules about what goes into their children's bodies. What if you saw Grandma--or anyone else for that matter--putting a refined oil product into the tank of your new automobile? Well you would be absolutely without a doubt mad as heck, and probably have to tow your car to a mechanic to have the engine cleaned out to keep it from being ruined! All fuel is not created equal!

So what about little Johnny's engine? What about his internal organs, his brain cells, his huge chances of becoming stricken with childhood leukemia (which is exploding in America), a child diabetic, or later in life having cancer, heart disease or Alzheimer's? And more likely than not, he may be having attention deficit problems that are absolutely caused from processed foods.

If your child has an attention deficit problem then you should give this plan a try: throw away all refined processed foods and sugars in your house and feed them only real unrefined foods. Then see what happens next. They may complain and refuse the healthy choices at first, but within a few days they will be hungry enough to eat real foods. I think you will be pleasantly surprised at the results.

You don't actually believe for one second that doctors have ever cured even one child in history by letting them stay on sugars and processed foods, do you? The answer most doctors give is to just pump their fragile little sick bodies full of horribly dangerous drugs--drugs that allow uncontrollable insulin levels from sugary foods to be masked. Doctors prescribe children what they call child-safe antidepressants--meds that turn your child into a zombie, not to mention becoming a prescription drug addict for life. GIVE ME A BREAK, FOLKS!

Dr. Leon Eisenberg (1922--2009) was a famous American child psychiatrist, first in his field of expertise in child psychiatry and autism. For decades he was considered the highest accredited expert on child behavioral and mental problems. No one knew more than Eisenberg about the (so-called) ADHD mental health issue. A 2012 article from the German publication 'Der Spiegel' describes an interview that Dr. Eisenberg gave seven months before his death in which he said that "ADHD is a prime example of a fabricated disease". He claimed the consideration of genetic predisposition to ADHD is totally overrated, and that "instead of prescribing dangerous medications, doctors should first determine if there are any psychosocial problems that could actually lead to any such behavior problems". In other words, don't dope-up little four year-old Susie to a lifetime of medication and living in the shadow of a tainted diagnosis just because she's anxious and full of energy while visiting the doctors office. Change her diet!

We do love our children more than that, don't we? Of course we do. We have just been marketed to and lied to for decades. We have trusted our government, our doctors, our drug companies, and our food processors to take care of us. Well guess what? Unfortunately, it has turned out that they not only didn't and don't take care of us, but they have seriously caused the ruined health of generations of the American people. Politicians, drug companies, and food refineries have made billions of dollars lying to us for their own personal gain. That's why I say: when it comes to your health and welfare, always go with your heart and just eat like our ancestors did a few hundred years ago.

I can almost remember the day, the hour and the second like it was yesterday, I was eight-years old and riding bicycles with my cousin Mark. As we ventured out of his Glendale, Arizona neighborhood, all of a sudden I realized I was coasting through a convenience store parking lot, then another, and another--and they seemed to never end! And again, let me remind you that in 1965, Knoxville, Tennessee was a small town with mostly mom-and-pop stores, and I had never seen or known of convenience stores in all my wildest imagination. As I begged my cousin to stop at this store, I remember him telling me that he had no money. But I was so anxious (addicted) and just wanted to see what one looked like inside. I begged him to stop. I told him not to worry that I always had (drug/sugar) money with me. I probably only had 50 cents in my pocket at the time, but that was plenty enough for me to gain entrance into one of those what I now call 'poison centers'.

Once I was inside, I almost went into a coma just looking at 2000 square feet of candy, donuts, chips, jerky, and of course a dozen different flavors of Slurpees. When the cashier asked if that was all, I remember thinking I had died and gone to heaven. I had never seen a Slurpee machine before that day, and I was instantly addicted. Arizona was a much larger test market for processed refined foods than the quaint and quiet little East Tennessee town I came from--and it had many more flavors of sugary treats to choose from than I had ever seen in my life. As each vacation passed, I became wiser. I prepared in advance by saving hard-earned money just to pay for my fix while on the family vacation.

While many of you might say that we all ate lots of candy as kids, it was truly a horrific addiction in my case. All I thought about on these vacations (after arriving in Phoenix and hugging my grandparents) was finding a way to get to a convenience store (poison center) as fast as possible. That usually involved telling my parents that I was going outside to play, only to escape to a four-lane very busy main highway three blocks away--looking for my fix. After filling my pockets with candy, I would hurry back to my grandparents house and find my parents panicking about where I had gone. And year after year I told them I was playing in the alley behind the house. I would lie with a sorrowful face just as a drug addict would.

I hope these stories are amusing and also inspirational, but I also hope and pray that your children are protected from the dangers I put myself through--not to mention the horrible health problems that followed me through five decades of eating processed refined sugars in every possible form, as well as foods that were cooked with highly inflammatory cell-killing substances. As you read this book, please do not feel sorry for me, because there is a fairly good chance that you and your children are eating just the same way that I did and simply just don't realize what it's doing to you.

On our annual western vacations we would always save a night to eat at a local famous steakhouse that offered a 32-ounce steak for free--if you could eat all of it. It was a challenge that everyone seemed to enjoy, and I desperately tried to do this more than once (despite the fact I wasn't picking up the tab). I didn't understand as a kid that that juicy steak was actually bad for my health. The 32-ounce steak that I was bloating myself on was not from the healthy cows that I would see grazing on beautiful green grass hillsides and valleys back in the beautiful hills and valleys of East Tennessee. Those 'eat it all for free' ones were actually cut from the animals I would see along the roadway in Texas and Oklahoma--standing by the tens of thousands shoulder to shoulder with their hides covered in animal feces because there wasn't even enough room to graze without laying in another animal's feces. Just go to your computer and simply type in the words 'feedlot cattle' and then prepare yourself for the terrible conditions that our daily grocery store food comes from in America. These cattle are fed huge amounts of corn and soybean meal, then pumped full of antibiotics, growth hormones, estrogens and a slew of other disease-causing chemicals. They are also given weight-building products like white bread and candy just before slaughter. And yes I said candy. Feedlot operators are allowed (by the law they created) to feed animals anything that is considered a food product. These products are usually machine damaged during processing and are sold to mega animal operations at a small price in order to fatten the animals just before slaughter. Do the math folks. MORE WEIGHT = MORE MONEY!!

A ruminant animal usually has a neutral PH and is designed by it's creator to eat a diet of grass. Cattle did not evolve onto this earth to eat grains (sugars), corn, and drugs like these feedlot cattle are being fed. Corn sickens cattle, bloats their stomachs, and makes them very acidic, which allows diseases and E.coli to develop. Are you starting to get the picture? A grass-fed cow grazing on pure grass and clover rarely has to have antibiotics and ends up on the dinner table as a pure natural (healing) wholesome real protein source. Compare that to a cow that was fed sugar and drugs and most likely was in poor health at the time of slaughter. It is a fact that a stressed (diseased) animal is not a healthy animal and therefore not something that you would want to put on your dinner table for your family.

Some folks often say things like "all fats are the same", and of course my immediate answer is "oh no they are not". The fat ingested from a healthy grass-fed animal helps regulate things in your body such as hormone balance, brain cell growth, thyroid function, muscle growth and healthy levels of HDL good cholesterol--just to mention a few. Something as simple as knowing where your steak comes from could make a huge difference in a healthy lifestyle. I recommend not consuming what I call chemical cows that could make you suffer from things like bad cholesterol, heart disease, cancer, oxidized arteries, poor thyroid conditions and diabetes. Do you really think it's worth the risk to feed your family anything besides pure healthy grass-fed beef?

The next time you take your children out for fast-food burgers might be the best time to look at the feedlot internet sites. If you're smart you'll gather up your children, load them in the car and drive away from fast-food as fast as you can--without ever looking back. The best gift you can ever give your child is to feed them only grass-fed meat and dairy, natural farm eggs and poultry, organic vegetables and fruits, and never feed them anything that is sold in a can, box or any refined processed product. I believe this is much more important than any other form of education.

Okay before all of you parents and scholars throw your books at me, just remember that the facts prove it's impossible to educate a sugared-up attention deficit child. If you have doubts then try it both ways and I bet I know who wins: no, not me. You and your children win big. If you think what I am saying is anything but the truth, then explain to me why 19% of American children are diagnosed with attention deficit while in France--where children eat a diet similar to John Rankin's Way, the attention deficit rate is diagnosed at only 0.4%. It's not a phenomenon. You do the math, folks.

I often talk to people who tell me that it costs way too much to feed their family with real foods. I certainly can see where this is a concern to them. But then more often than not, they tell me about the ice cream, crackers, chips, dip, candy and frozen dinners that they just can't live without. Then I tell them to stop even before they finish with their terrible blood-clotting, cancer-causing list. I challenge each of you to look at your weekly food budget and then buy only all natural products without the refined processed foods. Then compare how much you spend. If you cannot do this for just two consecutive weeks then it is almost a sure thing that you are also chemically addicted--just as I was.

Just remember some very important factors here: I am not trying to point you out as a health loser. My sincere passion is to help you become a health winner. It is my heart's desire to share with you the truth and things I have learned about the healing powers of real food. I am telling you about the origins of my addiction and a few of the problems it created for me. All of my life I have been a great salesman and a master at convincing others of my passions. The only difference between a con artist and me is that I can only try to convince others of things that are real and that I truly believe to be the truth. It is solely my passion and true intent to help you by educating you and your loved ones, by sharing what I've learned from a lifetime of study, prayer, and most of all my very interesting personal experiences

In today's world everywhere you look there's an article about superfoods. It never ceases to amaze me that in this day and time, most folks don't even know what real food is. You would be surprised at how many people ask me daily what I mean when I mention real food. Obviously with decades of fake marketing, it's no fault of their own. All real food is superfood. It's no mystery or rocket science. It's just old-fashioned naturally created God-given food! But refineries and conspiring men have made it possible through marketing and media to change the minds of good people to the point that we no longer have natural common sense knowledge of what real food is. I often tell folks to simply eat like our ancestors did, and they respond by saying, "Yes John, like in the 1930's or 1940's." No. Think again.

Large food refineries were well established in the early and mid-19th century in America, so our food has been--or has had the potential to be--tampered with for quite some time now. Processed sugar refineries have been producing their poison around the world for approximately five-hundred years. As we shop for food to feed our families, we must always be suspicious of what is in the packages and make smart choices about what we bring home to our dinner table. Do you think it's just a coincidence that America is one of the sickest countries in the world, even though we are one of the most educated with the best healthcare systems in all of the industrialized countries? Educated in what? Obviously not in the things that matter the most for our natural welfare.

To give you an example, just look at places like Okinawa where people often live to be over one-hundred years old. There are more centenarians there than anywhere in the world. Although these areas are very poor in financial wealth with unfavorable health care, the average person is not malnourished and sad, but instead very happy and healthy. They are among the healthiest people on earth. What do they do differently than we do? You might get tired of me saying this, but they eat all natural grass-fed meat, fish, eggs from natural free-range chickens, vegetables out of their own gardens, raw unpasteurized milk and cheese, and an abundant amount of unsprayed, unsulfured, non-irradiated fruits, vegetables. nuts and seeds--just like the American family did in the 18th century. We need only to take a closer look at those countries that we thought were so poor and where we felt sorry for their peoples. Believe me when I say the words, don't feel sorry for them but only for ourselves.

HEALED BY FARM
CHAPTER FIVE

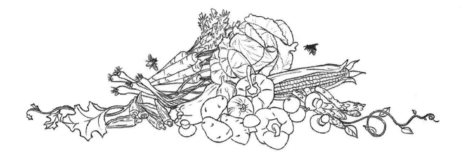

BIG BOX STORES

"The processed and refined foods that the food companies are marketing to you and your young children have been proven through thousands of studies to cause almost every poor health condition out there."

Sandwiches made with packaged meats and cheeses were not the only thing coming to my small hometown in the mid-1960's. The larger grocery store chains were starting to show up in town, and I vividly remember when the first big box grocery store opened up within bicycle-range of my house. Besides the extra large bag of popcorn that I purchased there daily (which was made with oxidized inflammatory trans fat oils and soaked in inflammatory refined processed sodium), I found something new and exciting added to my life. With the arrival of these stores, I was able to instantly improve my marketing skills with items that got me out of the cherry cough drop business.

At first thought you might think this was a good thing, but it was actually anything but good. With the coming of these new stores in town, I was able to purchase multiples of varieties of candy bars in large packages at just a fraction of the cost I was paying for them at the old mom-and-pop stores! I remember just how wonderful it was to purchase twenty-five candy bars all at once in one package for such a small price. Big box stores changed my life as they enabled me to advance my addiction a long way from climbing the cabinets and stealing my father's jelly beans.

When I was in elementary school, kids didn't carry backpacks and I didn't carry a lunchbox. I bought school lunches, so you can just imagine how hard it was to smuggle a dozen or more monster chocolate candy bars out of the house in my mother's presence, onto the school bus with my older siblings, and into a fourth grade classroom--past my teacher--all without anyone noticing! Well that's not exactly true: my faithful customers--to whom I had been selling sugar since the first grade--were well aware of what I daily carried to school stuffed into my clothing.

I started off in the first grade earning pennies from my friends, and by the fourth grade I was earning dimes and quarters from them. I was the largest candy (drug) dealer in my grade level and probably in the entire school. During these school years, none of the other kids ever exposed my little business venture to our teachers. And why would they? They were addicted to the same attention-deficit-causing, teeth-rotting, stomach ache-causing, inflammatory processed and refined corn sugars that I was addicted to! If we had any idea what these 'treats' were doing to our health, you would think we would have just run away from this stuff. We probably would have except for just a couple of things that just happened to get into our way.

The first thing, as I mentioned before, is that recent university studies are proving that processed and refined sugars (including high fructose corn syrup) are eight times more addictive than cocaine. The second thing is the fact that hundreds of millions of dollars are spent annually on advertising and conspiring marketing schemes which target small children, in hopes they or their parents will purchase their (disease-causing) products. It's no secret about where the food companies position candy at the store checkout lines: eye level to the children. In my opinion the food companies are considered and should be called predators--health predators that is. But either way that title is appropriate, and if you look up the definition of 'predator' it will explain that it is something that stalks, attacks, and then eventually kills its victims. Well friends, I guess that terminology is well put because the processed and refined foods that the food companies are marketing to you and your young children have been proven through thousands of studies to cause almost every poor health condition out there: diabetes, cancer, heart disease, Alzheimer's, thyroid failure and an array of others. So PLEASE PLEASE PLEASE don't believe for one second that the soda you drink, the bag of chips you eat, or even the adulterated meat and dairy that you feed your family may or may not hurt you. IT WILL.

I think it would totally shock you if you really knew how many people in this country are diabetics. No, these people are not just strangers or someone that you see in the doctor's office waiting room. These folks are you, your spouses, your close friends and most sadly your own precious children. Unfortunately, there are over twenty-five million people in the United States with type II diabetes and over one-million children with type I diabetes (twenty-thousand per state), and that number is skyrocketing every day. Many more of your friends than you can imagine have this horrific disease--most of them just do not announce their illnesses.

Just take a look around you while you're sitting in church, at the mall or even the gym. When you see someone that is several sizes larger than a normal person is supposed to be, or the explosion in the number of obese folks riding around the stores on electric trikes, the odds are very much in favor that they are

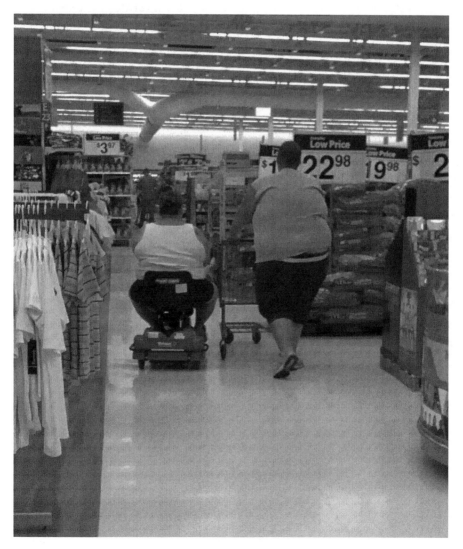

diabetics. Again, not judging but just observing so I can better help you with your health. Fifty years ago we did not have a hundred handicap parking spaces and a store full of unfortunate three-hundred and fifty pound folks cruising around the aisles on electric carts.

So what's the deal? First of all let me make myself very clear that in no way would I ever make fun of unhealthy overweight people. I would also advise you to never judge someone for their bad decisions or misfortunes in life. We need only to reach out to these people and inspire and teach them how to change their health in order to improve the quality of their lives. Folks, America is in trouble and we need each other. Unfortunately 99.9% of these handicapped overweight sick people have one thing in common: they made unwise choices during their lifetime. But most disturbing is the very true fact that the giant (fake food) companies have misled them with total lies about the safety of their foods, while at the same time falsifying the scientific data that actually proves most refined processed foods cause inflammation and oxidation in your bodies. INFLAMMATION = EXCESS BODY FAT, CANCER, CLOGGED ARTERIES and so much more.

I just want to laugh myself silly every time I read an article of a so-called scientific study by a major university that tries to convince us that just a small amount of refined processed sugar won't hurt us or is actually good for us. Some studies suggest that just a few grams of sugar per day won't hurt us at all.

WRONG AGAIN! Put a small amount of crack cocaine in your mouth and see what happens. What is the difference? None. They both hook you forever and they both will eventually ruin your health and probably take your life.

Now don't get me wrong. There are some honest universities doing honest studies out there--just not many. And there are way too many of these studies that are bought and paid for by giant fake food producers. It's happening every day in our country. Giant fake food companies are donating millions of dollars to build new research centers on campuses all over America. In return, these universities agree to let the giant fake food producers put their professor of choice in charge of the classroom curriculum, teaching false data to conspire and fool everyone from health care providers to consumers.

If this sounds somewhat fanatical and hard to believe, well it's anything but that. Actually it is very much the truth about what is happening in our world every day of our lives. Just click online and look up who is on the board of trustees at that institution who also works for one or more of the major food companies. Check out the list of donations coming to that institution from those same food companies. Once again you will be shocked by what you learn, and we haven't even yet touched on the epidemic of paybacks to politicians and doctors by pharmaceutical companies. It's bad enough when a politician or someone of authority takes a bribe to let something such as a new road contract go to a friend, and then it's another thing when they take a bribe from the food or drug industry that will ensure a new product on your supermarket shelves that will sicken you and your children if you eat it. In this case it becomes personal.

As parents, we all have defended our children when another neighborhood parent accuses little Johnny of something he didn't do or a teacher didn't treat him just the way you think they should. You always come to your children's rescue. How would you feel if you just found out that someone was trying to poison your child? You would want to have that person put away for a very long time. Well guess what? That terrible person could very well be you. And no, you're not a terrible parent. It's just that you are being lied to and taken advantage of by the mega giant fake food company's marketing schemes to addict you, just as I was before I learned about their conspiring ways.

If your family's breakfast comes out of a box, has more than three ingredients, or has the word 'fortified' on the label, chances are it isn't real food at all. It may be cooked with oxidized trans fat oils, loaded with things like monosodium glutamate (usually disguised with dozens of confusing names meant to deceive you), bleached white genetically-modified flour, and contain a list of chemicals that you could make rat poison with. Oh that's right--studies show that these ingredients do kill rats in laboratory studies. It's these same chemicals that are destroying your gut bacteria and causing stomach problems that you assume are gluten or celiac problems, among other distresses. I will talk about those problems later in the book.

When you pick up a box of cereal or other product in the store and you see those big bold letters that say the product is fortified with vitamins, you should put it back on the shelf and run away from it as fast as you can. Now you might think that sounds like a silly thing to do when the product is simply touting that it has extra vitamins. You will want to know that when these food products are milled, processed and mixed with oxidized hydrogenated oils and dangerous chemicals and then cooked at extreme heat, they lose almost all of their mineral and vitamin composition. So basically almost 100% of the nutrients of that so-called food are destroyed in the high heat cooking process, and then the food scientist adds about 10% of a dangerous synthetic version of vitamins back to the mix to call it fortified--when all the while they have you believing that their product has 110% of a great and nutritious vitamin source.

In a newly released study by the Environmental Working Group (EWG), we learn that almost 50% of children in the United States age eight and younger eat potentially harmful amounts of vitamin A, zinc, and niacin from excessive food for- tification and vitamin supplements. Too much vitamin A can and is causing liver damage, bone abnormalities, and a host of other horrific problems like abnormalities in the fetus during pregnancy. Funny thing though, the report also confirmed that excessive vitamin A from natural real foods such as carrots and pumpkin is considered totally safe for kids--with no side effects--thus my accurate description of dangerous for synthetic vitamin infusions.

Is it all starting to make sense, folks? All natural real food equals a great quality life without sickness, while man-made refined, processed foods equal a lifetime of sickness and even premature death! Now here is the funniest thing you will hear all day. Just after this report came out, one of the leading cereal manufacturers came out with this quote: "We at the cereal company are concerned with this report and that a great deal of nutrition for children comes from ready to eat cereals". I haven't stopped laughing at this spokesman and the cereal company's response yet. And yes, the cereal company should be concerned--with their profits that is. As we learn more about these dangerous products and quit buying them, then and only then will these huge fake food producers stop lying to us about their harmful products for the sake of big profits for their shareholders.

Wait just a minute, did I say shareholders? You might just want to check with your stockbroker and take a look into your own portfolio to see if you are actually supporting the very food processing companies that are sickening your own families with their toxic so-called foods. I equate this to buying stock in a foreign military that is attacking our homeland! There are literally thousands of good growth company stocks available without supporting cancer, diabetes, heart disease and a slew of other illnesses.

Additionally, here is a little known fact that should open your eyes: our very own health insurance companies buy stock in fast food chains all over the world. Now at first thought that just doesn't make much sense. They should want us to stay healthy and not eat fast food in order to keep healthcare costs down, right? That shows us as a nation how addicted we are to this kind of poisonous food that our healthcare providers would insure us and hope that we stay healthy--but then bet against us that we won't. They don't have much confidence in us, and for good reason. Wouldn't it be great if all of us could prove them wrong as we eat real food again and stop being the sickest nation in the world?

HEALED BY FARM
CHAPTER SIX

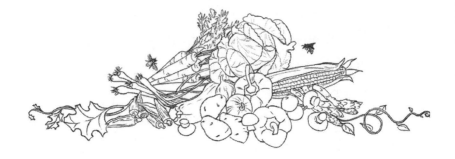

ROAD TO DISASTER

"A human body that consumes processed refined sugar also has acute inflammation in every cell and organ tissue, which is an open invitation to almost every disease we have ever heard about."

By the time I was nine or ten years old, I was a master at selling everything from sugary products to bicycles. I often laugh
to myself when folks tell me they have worked ever since they
were sixteen years old. I started my own business at age five!
No, I'm not still selling candy, but while in Boy Scouts no other
scout in town could outsell me at door-to-door fundraisers. I
remember my scoutmaster asking me just how in the world I
could sell candy to every house in the neighborhood. Little did
he know (and would have been shocked if he knew) what I had
been doing daily for years.

In 1890, the diabetes rate was around three people per
100,000 population. Today there are about 10,000 diabetics
per 100,000 people living in America--one in ten. That is
a total increase of 9,997 per 100,000 people, and if that's
not enough to wake you up then we have a lot of work to do
here, folks.

In 1895, the obesity rate for white males in their fifties in
America was 3.4%. In 1976 the obesity rate for all of the U.S.
population had jumped to 15%. By 2010, 35.7% of adults and
17% of children in the United States were obese.

Let me backup and give you a little history lesson on sugar
and associated health issues. The first refined sugar appeared
in Europe in the year 1100, and was so expensive and sought
after that it was called white gold. America's current fascina-
tion with this white poison started after the discovery of this
continent by Christopher Columbus. They found the islands

of the Caribbean to be the perfect place to grow sugarcane. In the mid-15th century men were taken from Africa and sold as slaves to work the sugarcane fields in Spain. The first sugar refinery opened in Germany in 1537, and since that very day has been the cause of increased horrific health problems and deaths.

In 1493, Queen Isabella ordered Columbus to ship sugarcane back to England after which sugar refineries started up there. It was during this period of time that people began succumbing to the sugar addiction. In the year 1560, Charles V of Spain placed vast taxes on sugar. He built huge palaces with these taxes from human slave labor. In my own words, I definitely call him a conspiring evil man.

During the next century the sugar industry grew so fast that the British passed the navigation act of 1660 to prevent any nation or port other than their own from receiving the (newly addictive) substance. By 1662, Britain was importing 16 million pounds of sugarcane per year. Through history (not my theory) we have learned that in 1665, just a few years after refined sugar was introduced, approximately 68,000 people died in London from the bubonic plague. What most of us have not learned from our history lessons (and I'm assuming conspiring men left it out) is the very true fact that most people who lived at this time without processed sugar (white gold) escaped harm from that plague.

In 1674, less than ten years later, Thomas Willis, a member

of the college of physicians, discovered the first case of diabetes. Surely refined processed sugar didn't have anything to do with it. OF COURSE IT DID!!! Read and learn and be smart people. So then if we are so smart and educated, why can't we just put this white poison down and simply walk away from it? It's that little word I've spoken about many times over and over--ADDICTION. Now let me add three more words, YES YOU ARE!!! And once again let me be clear that I am not pointing you out as a health loser. You are just someone who--like most Americans--needs a little help with the how-to, and it is my life destiny to be that help for as many people as possible before I leave this God-given beautiful earth.

So since sugar is proven to be eight times more addictive than cocaine, do the math folks: a sugar addiction is like taking the drug cocaine and mixing an ingredient to it that makes it eight times stronger than its original composition, then eat it daily for a lifetime. It's no wonder that great palaces were built from the introduction of the refining process from the once innocent and somewhat healthy sugarcane plant.

By 1770, Britain was importing twenty million pounds of sugar per year. In that same year tuberculosis increased dramatically in that and other countries where such large amounts of sugar were consumed. I'm not claiming sugar directly caused these diseases, but it's not a coincidence the majority of the population who didn't get sick are the same people who didn't eat the poison. At that time in history only the affluent people could afford the white gold and the poor could not, and the poor people did not get these deadly diseases. That's not my theory--history absolutely proves it. My theory is that it is an absolute fact, a human body that consumes processed refined sugar also has acute inflammation in every cell and organ tissue, which is an open invitation to almost every disease we have ever heard about.

It never ceases to amaze me that in this modern world our so-called trusted health officials along with our heart and cancer associations are still covering up or lying to us about the safety of our food. What's in it for them you say? Greed, money, and power, (surely not!) The next time you eat out at a restaurant or more particularly your local sandwich shops, take notice of the heart-healthy logo next to items on the menu. Heart-healthy from what? Well it couldn't be from all of the refined inflammatory salt, MSG, sugar, and nitrates in the meat (that university studies absolutely prove will cause heart disease and cancer). Nope, not that.

Maybe it's the bleached flour bread loaded with stomach health killing chemicals and even more inflammatory salt, sugar and MSG--not to mention the genetically modified wheat. Nope, not heart-healthy either.

Maybe it's the salad dressing that is made from hydrogenated oils, MSG, sugar and an enormous amount of refined inflammatory sodium and preservatives. Nope, not heart healthy either.

What is it in the sandwiches that our heart association thinks is so heart-healthy? Is it the lettuce that is packed in sulfite (chlorine) preservatives? Nope, not that. Maybe they are just skipping over all of these highly inflammatory refined products that will cause disease to your body and just assuming that the lettuce and pepper on your sandwich is heart-healthy. I think I would just eat that part and throw the rest of the sandwich away--except for the fact that if they are being sold at most restaurants, they are probably mass grown with enormous amounts of dangerous chemicals (crop dusting) with quite a large dose of herbicides and pesticides.

I've only mentioned a short list of the ingredients that our trusted heart associations will stamp with their approval. Why do they do this, you ask? I cannot answer that question. But I do know for a fact that millions and millions of dollars are regularly donated to the heart associations from fast food restaurant chains--for their stamp of approval? Again, do the math folks.

I honestly cannot quit laughing at the fact that the heart associations actually rate these foods on their fat content alone and not on the hydrogenated oils, sugar, nitrates, MSG, and refined sodium (that modern day science absolutely proves is the real cause of disease in America and now around the world as well). It is no coincidence that the good people of China have recently started becoming fat and sick for the first time in history. And one guess what just showed up in their country for the first time in history. Yep, AMERICAN FAST FOOD RESTAURANTS!! It is widely known that these products and chemicals cause inflammation in every cell in our body, which then causes our good HDL cholesterol to drop to unhealthy levels while our LDL bad cholesterol particles become dense and tiny and cause hardening of the arteries and even death.

You will want to know that there are some vital studies currently being done at major universities such as UCLA, proving that cancer cells die when we reduce inflammation. These promising studies are also showing that by reducing inflammation, Alzheimer's disease is quite possibly reversed. How could that be you might ask? Because we have been led to believe that only another drug therapy could possibly save us from Alzheimer's and that we need more funding to study it.

These are the facts folks: REAL FOOD HEALS. Your body has to have healthy fats (including cholesterol) in your diet to build brain cells and to regulate hormone and thyroid function. And here's the best news: healthy fats actually lower inflammation.

Now hold the shopping cart just a minute. Don't go out to your local grocery store tomorrow and buy out the meat and dairy section just yet. There's a lot more for me to explain so that you shop at the right stores and farmers' markets to get the healthiest products. Deceptive fake food marketing wants to sell you items that contain dangerous hidden ingredients. I want you to get educated first and then make wise choices accordingly.

I personally eat a moderate amount of red meat, fish, pork, and poultry, natural free-range eggs, and a fairly good serving of dairy from raw unpasteurized milk, including kefir, cheese, yogurt and butter. At a recent appointment, my doctor was reading my blood lipid panel results to me. He was very impressed with my results in raising my good HDL cholesterol with a 61% increase in just over six months. He was also amazed at the fact that I lowered my C-Reactive Protein (a test for inflammation level) to basically zero, which results are nearly nonexistent in our society. That low score just never happens. He then acknowledged that what I had done was absolutely wonderful and mostly unheard of in America, congratulating me on my results.

Then in the same breath this doctor told me to be very careful because American studies showed that some of the things I was eating proved to be harmful! I just looked at him like a deer in the headlights! Here I sat looking at a blood lipid test that most men my age (or any age) would kill for! And I was being told to be careful with what I had been eating? My immediate response to him was this: "You know, Doc, you are certainly right. American studies do show that these fats and foods that I'm eating can be harmful to your health. On the other hand, the same studies in European and Asian countries (that have been done exactly like the American studies for 60 years) reveal polar opposite effects than the American studies

while using the same number of people, gender, age etc."
He agreed.

So then we must ask ourselves, "Which country is cheating on their tests and not telling the truth?" Both studies are actually telling the truth. The simple difference is that the American studies have been using subjects who eat what I would like to refer to as chemical animals from feedlots--animals that eat a diet consisting only of genetically modified corn and soybean meal, and everything from white bread to old gummy bears--with a dose of antibiotics and growth hormones. The American human studies on egg consumption are examined with what I call factory eggs that are produced with GMO grains, antibiotics, growth hormones and other dangerous drugs, and are produced in dark chicken houses under unsanitary, diseased conditions. As for American human studies on consuming dairy products, the so-called clinical trials have been done with subjects consuming pasteurized and homogenized dairy. Science absolutely proves that the extreme heat from pasteurization almost certainly cooks out most minerals and vitamins in the chemically induced water thinning process.

Now let's travel over to some of the European, Asian and Middle Eastern countries whose claims show that all these same foods will actually heal your body and turn you into a healthy human being! Their studies have been done using grass-fed animals that were not fed sugar by-products with added growth hormones and antibiotics. The test subjects in these countries were fed eggs from chickens that naturally ate grass, seeds, bugs and worms like nature intended (which creates up to 200% more omega-3 fatty acids and a much superior source of protein, not to mention the exquisite taste). As for the dairy studies, they use blood test results from subjects who consume raw grass-fed milk, cheese, butter and yogurt. These are exactly the kinds of natural foods that my family and I consume on a daily basis.

With this kind of scientific data and open records available to us, our government agencies, cancer and heart associations, and food and drug companies still deny that these studies are true and that these products will actually heal you from disease. At the very same time our governmental agencies are telling us not to consume healthy grass-fed raw dairy products, raw milk vending machines are being installed around Europe. How could this be, you might ask?

Well let me just say this: it's a well-known fact that politicians and some folks at our governmental agencies are very cozy with big agriculture in America. Lobbying is big business in our country. How do I know for sure that eating real meat and dairy with natural omega-3 fats, linoleic and conjugated acids will actually heal your body? "My blood tests don't lie! Body fat and inflammation markers don't either". In other words, my blood tests prove it. It's not just a coincidence, folks, that my family, friends, and acquaintances who eat identically to my all-natural plan just happen to have perfect or near perfect blood lipid panels too. It's Mother Nature's plan-- and it works.

And now before we go much farther slamming doctors, just let me tell you how understanding my doctors are and what great friends we have become. They are not what I would call 'pill-pushers', and they support my healthy living lifestyle 100%. If this country had more doctors like them who are actually willing to learn and heal their patients, then we would be a much healthier nation. I would also like to thank all the necessary emergency docs and surgeons who have patched my body back together after a lifetime of active adventures that some would call more like stuntman activities.

As for the thousands of fairytale American studies, mostly done by conspiring food companies and their own employed scientists, and the articles that claim raw whole dairy is dangerous and clogs arteries and will make you fat--then just hold on a minute while I stop laughing again. For those of you who eat low-fat dairy (if with any fat at all), with very little meat and no fibrous bread, I have two questions for you: "How many diets have you been on and how is it working out for you?" I'm assuming it's not working very well or you wouldn't be reading this book.

If you are not eating healthy fats and fiber and are losing weight, then you are guaranteed to be malnourished and will have a higher body weight after your diet is over. Believe me, you can only starve yourself for a short period of time and your

blood tests will certainly tell on you. Almost all low-fat foods
are loaded with sugar and other dangerous chemicals that will
actually make you fat and inflamed. You will absolutely damage your health by eating these low-fat, chemical-laden foods.
It's just fake food folks. These dangerous chemicals create
immediate inflammation in your bodies when you eat them,
which in turn form free radicals that cause everything from
premature aging of your skin, thyroid failure, heart disease,
cancer, arthritis and certainly Alzheimer's disease. The only
sure and proven way to avoid or even cure these diseases is to
eat only anti-inflammatory real whole foods.

It is widely known that some people (especially women)
push dairy aside in fear of getting fat. The idea that real raw
unpasteurized dairy makes you fat and clogs your arteries
couldn't be further from the truth. In case you haven't noticed,
breast cancer rates have risen dramatically over the past few
decades as women have parked their dairy at the back of the
refrigerator. Good news ladies: many recent studies show scientific proof that women who have conjugated linoleic acid in
their bloodstream (CLA) have a 60-75% less chance of getting
breast cancer. Numerous studies are also proving CLA's are
causing mass weight loss in animal and human studies. Like
I've said for years, BODY FAT=INFLAMMATION=CANCER.
Get rid of the fat naturally and disease dies. I would take those
odds if I were you. And I'll give you one guess where these
CLA's come from? That's right girls: real grass-fed meat and

raw unpasteurized dairy from grass-fed animals.

I don't know about you, but I would just choose real steak and cheese any time over radiation, chemotherapy, and even death. Folks, there is absolutely no reason for you or your loved ones to suffer and die like this. As for the weight gain you think might happen if you eat natural real food, well guess what? When I mentioned the food studies between the different countries with polar opposite results, I wasn't just talking about blood test results.

Take a moment to observe what people look like in some of the European, Asian and Middle Eastern areas where they eat mostly raw natural foods. One thing is for certain--you won't see them dragging their butts around grocery stores on electric shopping carts! People in these whole-food-eating countries generally have a natural lean and healthy look, including their skin.

While the cholesterol scam is alive and well in America, with the drug companies setting the approved levels for what's healthy with blood results, other populations abroad allow their total cholesterol levels to be much higher. And for some reason they are much healthier with less disease! I'm almost certain by now that you are repeating the words "how, how, how"? Well I'll tell you how and then I'll keep telling you until you have healed yourself. The people in these other countries who eat only real natural foods--avoiding foods that cause inflammation--have excellent health.

The *French Paradox* is a catch phrase first used in the late 1980's that summarizes the apparently paradoxical observation that the French people have a relatively low incidence of coronary heart disease (CHD), while having a diet relatively rich in saturated fats. This is in apparent contradiction to the widely held belief that the high consumption of such fats is a risk factor for CHD. The paradox is that if the idea linking saturated fats to CHD is valid, the French ought to have a higher rate of CHD than comparable countries where the per capita consumption of such fats is lower.

The *French Paradox* implies two important possibilities. The first is that the hypothesis linking saturated fats to CHD is not completely valid (or entirely invalid). The second possibility is that the link between saturated fats and CHD is valid, but that some additional factor in the French diet or lifestyle (such as a glass of wine a day or a super-chill lifestyle) mitigates this risk—with the idea that if the truth of this factor can be identified, it can be incorporated into the diet and lifestyle of other countries, with the same lifesaving success observed in France. Both possibilities have brought considerable media interest, as well as some scientific research. This research suggests that the so-called *French Paradox* is attributed to the fact that the French people consume much more healthy saturated fats and have much higher total cholesterol levels, with much less coronary heart disease than Americans.

For most of my life I have studied people who have the same

goals I have. If things are working better for them than for me, then I would just simply follow their example and do things their way. I can write a dozen health books for you to study, but if you don't follow my example then you will never know if these things are true. Everything in life comes down to our choices, and right now you have a choice to make. You can choose to have your doctor give you another dangerous drug that you saw advertised on television that most certainly will not heal your body. Or you can stand in front of the mirror, take a deep breath, look at yourself, and decide to take charge of your own body. You can decide to take a few short weeks eating only what Mother Nature gives us and learn for yourself if this works. I believe that most pharmaceutical medicines do not heal--they only mask symptoms and perhaps buy time.

Take a look at your choice: eat delicious whole food and watch disease and excess body fat literally leave your body, or go to the hospital and let them stick needles in both arms being held in place with tape for days, taking your blood about 30 times while more hoses, wires and monitors are hooked to your body, all the while lying there for even more days before you're taken to surgery--where you will be pumped full of dangerous drugs, put unconscious, and then gutted open by a guy who is going to later tell you about all of the wonderful drugs that you will be taking the rest of your miserable life. I'm fairly certain I would just choose the real tasty food option if I were you! I did, and it worked for me.

You probably have discovered by now that I am totally black-and-white and some might even think I am somewhat intense. Then thanks, I'm doing my job. Most of us have read a lot of dietary advice--everything from low-fat is healthier to just a little sugar won't hurt you. If these things were even remotely true and actually worked, you wouldn't be desperately searching for the truth. Hopefully by now you have parked your last popsicle and are following my advice, telling your doctors that the rules are going to change, having them listen to your plan now. Who knows, you might even teach them something that will change their lives for the better. If they don't approve of what you are doing, FIRE THEM. You pay the bill, not them.

HEALED BY FARM
CHAPTER SEVEN

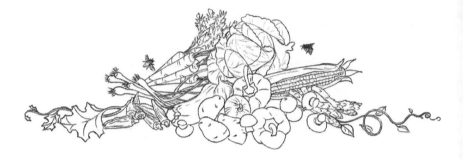

FIRST OBSERVATION

"...sugar poisoning will change your life in the blink of an eye--just like it did mine, over and over."

The years just can't roll by fast enough when you are a child. Waiting for my tenth birthday seemed to take forever. Not long before that day, I was across town visiting my paternal grandparents. My granddad had asked me to go for a walk around his neighborhood with him, and like always I was excited to go--knowing that we would as always walk past a small mom-and-pop store where I would certainly be awarded with candy and a soda with Granddad. (Of course I would have gone for a walk with anyone for candy and a soda)! Happy as I could be as Granddad and I left the store and resumed our walk back through the neighborhood, I didn't realize this would be our last walk together. I do remember however observing something that day that apparently was never a concern to me. I noticed that my granddad walked with a limp, and his right hand hung somewhat awkwardly at his side. He had always been that way, and as a nine year-old child I just always assumed old folks walked like that just because they were old. I learned later that he had suffered two strokes back about the time I was born, and apparently back then no one thought that a small child needed to know that kind of medical information.

My grandparents both grew up on farms and knew the importance of fresh farm food. But as the years passed, they had no idea what was happening to their bodies from the modern-day processed food that was being introduced into their lives. They had obviously become addicted to refined process sugars, as has almost all mankind for hundreds of years.

As I sat drinking a soda with my granddad and observing his worn out body, I had no clue what had made him that way. Not long after that day--less than four months after my 10th birthday, something went tragically wrong. My grandparents were traveling to their little farm just outside of town driving their little blue 1964 Ford Fairlane--without seatbelts--when my granddad suddenly and without warning suffered his third stroke.

Several witnesses at the scene told us of the valiant effort my grandfather made trying to stay in the lane just before they plowed head on into a power pole. The horrific crash hurled my sweet little grandmother into the windshield, killing her instantly. My granddad wasn't so lucky. His crumpled bleeding body lay lifeless at the scene in twisted metal and broken glass with almost every bone broken from his cheeks to his toes while nearly bleeding to death. The paramedic's report stated he had no detectable heart rate and not enough blood in his body for a human to survive, not to mention he was also in the middle of suffering his third horrific stroke.

Between the paramedics and the hospital ER doctors, they tried their best to pronounce my granddad dead, but he refused to die. The following weeks and months for him were horrendous, and let me just say to those of us who have minor afflictions in life, be so grateful and thank God daily. The very painful next chapter of my granddad's life (and mine) was a lesson that cannot be taught unless you actually live it. Nowadays I often wonder who this lesson was for, him or I. The next few months brought such misery not only to him but to our entire family. Remember folks, I now know that these life sobering events were solely caused from inflammatory processed sugars that my granddad enjoyed so much.

Week after week, the doctors continually gave him only hours to live. However after much physical and mental rehab, we thought he had the battle won. But I didn't win any battle. The reality was difficult for me. In the months and years following, I was given a lot of knowledge, understanding, and character building--some of the best lessons in my life.

Seat belts were not standard in cars in those days, and my father had bought some for them and had planned to install them in my grandparent's car before the accident. Thus he carried a lot of blame for the death of his mother and his crippled father, even though it certainly was not his fault nor predictable by anyone. The unrelenting guilt caused my father to fall into alcoholism to hide his deep depression. His alcohol dependence devastated our family for many years, and as a young man I had feelings of hatred toward my father for what he had become. Later in life, when I realized all of the suffering and pain that he endured in his life, I forgave my father. And as the years went by, he forgave himself as well and put things back together as best he could.

When my granddad was eventually released from the hospital, he came to live with us. We hired a maid/nurse who took

care of him each day, staying only until the school bus stopped
in front of our house and let me off. Yep, that's what I said--
until the school bus stopped. The moment I walked in the door
was the very moment the nurse walked out the door. My mom
was usually helping run my father's business, and my four
siblings were heading from school to jobs or for some other
reason wouldn't be home for at least another hour. Now picture this: you're barely eleven years old and the first one home
from school, a stack of newspapers sitting on a store sidewalk
waiting on you two miles away, a big collie scratching at the
door waiting to be fed, Mrs Johnson on the phone needing for
you to come over and mow her yard, all while my half-para-
lyzed broken down granddad was motioning and mumbling
to me that his urinal had overflowed and was spilling onto the
bed. Yes folks, this was a daily experience I wouldn't wish on
any eleven year-old.

But that's not really what I learned from this experience at
such a young age. I learned to be a caregiver as well as a thing
or two about love, discipline and respect. During the years
my granddad lived with us, my search for something began. I
did not know at that time what I was searching for, but I was
starting to connect the dots and realize something just wasn't
adding up. I vividly remember many times sharing my candy
with granddad as I wiped the slobber from his chin and the
urine from his body--all the while wondering why my sweet
little grandmother was dead and my granddad was a crippled

man who could barely mumble his words at best.

For the three years he lived with us and during his final three years in a nursing home, I often stood over Granddad wondering what was the difference between him and my other perfectly healthy grandparents living in Arizona. It was at that time in my life that I gained great respect for many older relatives and family friends who were in their 80's and 90's and still driving around and working their farms like they were decades younger. I knew something was different between these two sets of grandparents, but as a young teen I just couldn't quite put my finger on it. During these times of wondering what happened, and while continuing to share my candy with my granddad, little did I realize that I was going down the exact same road--the sugar road. I was setting myself up for a life like his. I was also blindsided by the fact that my father was traveling the same road and would arrive there before me. NO, NO, NO! Surely God was not going to put me through this twice in my lifetime? How could He do such a thing. Well, He did. And He did it to me more than twice. As I look back down that road of sadness in my life, I surely don't blame God for anything. I do however praise God for all of the knowledge, wisdom and understanding that He has given me which has finally allowed me to connect the dots. Hopefully connecting these dots will allow me to not only help my family but also others who struggle with the same addiction in their lives.

By now some of you are probably having doubts that something as simple as sugar can possibly be the cause of all of the horrific things that I have just described. After all, it's just sugar and everyone eats it, right? No, actually healthy folks who don't have diabetes, heart and thyroid disease, Alzheimer's and cancer don't eat processed sugar. And to all of you who say the words "I eat it and it doesn't hurt me," then you need to keep looking over your shoulder because it will slowly creep up on you. And like the poison it is, sugar poisoning will change your life and that of your family in the blink of an eye--just like it did mine, over and over.

The average one to three year-old American child consumes approximately 15 teaspoons of sugar per day. Regardless if you think your child does or not, it's in their processed food. That equates to 105 teaspoons per week, 420 per month, and over 5000 per year. This is according to national statistics, and my guess is that the reality is much higher than that. Please don't be in denial. As parents, we need to simply quit feeding our babies fast food and processed refined poison.

Many of us say that we just can't find the time to cook healthy meals to feed our families. For those who think this way, I would strongly encourage you to visit a nearby hospital and take a slow walk through the children's ward. Take a look at Mommy and Daddy's precious little two year-old child without hair and with intravenous needles stuck in their arms while dangerous chemotherapy drugs circulate all through their sick little organs. Talk to his or her parents who spend 24/7 in that hospital room watching their child slowly die from something that possibly could have prevented in the first place. If only the mega giant fake food producers had not conspired and intentionally mislabeled food to begin with. Let me just say that the parents of these kinds of circumstances are not guilty of anything. They love their children. First they are misled by food companies that add ingredients known to be carcinogenic, and then these companies actually lie and manipulate the ingredient list and rename it something else. (The FDA and USDA usually allow this under some flimsy ruling that gives food companies a free pass to poison us). And why would they disguise the name of the ingredients in the first place if these ingredients don't hurt us? When you're not trying to hide something don't you usually just give all the facts as they are?

Another average statistic on American teenage children says they are getting an average of 34 teaspoons of sugar per day from consuming three sodas. I am guessing that teens are getting double that amount considering the vast amount of fast food and store-bought refined fake food that goes into their bodies. Oh, and let's not forget the dangerous energy drinks!

My own teenage years were anything but healthy. At sixteen years of age, I watched my granddad wilt away and die. And I still had no clue that I was getting closer to growing up just like him. Some of you who are familiar with the lyrics of the song "Cat's in the Cradle--I'm going to be just like you Dad".

When we listened to this song years ago, most of us were

totally unaware just how much we would grow up just like Dad.

The doctor's suggested diet for my granddad was the most foolish thing I had ever witnessed in my life, but of course how was an eleven year-old boy supposed to know that a full grown man could not survive on a piece of white bread toast with margarine, water, a sprig of lettuce and a piece of feedlot chicken the size of a quarter, with a handful of pills? Okay doctors--before you get mad and throw your prescription pads at me, let me say this: most of you spend years and countless dollars going to medical school to learn how to help sick patients. I sincerely applaud you for your efforts, but unfortunately all the education in the world has not kept you from drinking the same kool-aid as the very same folks you are trying to save. Some of you are in the medical profession for the money and some are in it to help people heal, to save lives and really make a difference. Wouldn't it be wonderful to be known as the doctor who actually healed patients and put their lives back together instead of the guy who just prescribed dangerous drugs to them until they died? If your true desire is to help people heal, then take my advice and take a step back from your 12-14 hour work day, take a deep breath and look in the mirror and make the best decision of your life: to do what you

set out to do in the beginning of your medical career. I challenge anyone in the medical field to stop being dictated to by
big pharma and the mega giant fake food industries. I know
from personal experience (I was there) that hospital-sponsored
cardiac rehab classes nationwide are still telling sick patients
to eat liquefied hydrogenated margarine made from genetically
modified vegetable oil and liver-wrecking artificial sweeteners
with aspartame. And just where do you think they learn this
fake so-called knowledge from? Remember when I mentioned
the mega giant food company sponsored research schools
being built on campuses nationwide? DO THE MATH FOLKS-
SHAME ON THEM !!!

The food shown here was given to a patient who just had a massive heart attack. The meal includes all of the things that will cause a heart attack in the first place like processed sugar, MSG, refined sodium and hydrogenated trans fat, just to name a few. So just why in the heck are the hospitals doing this?

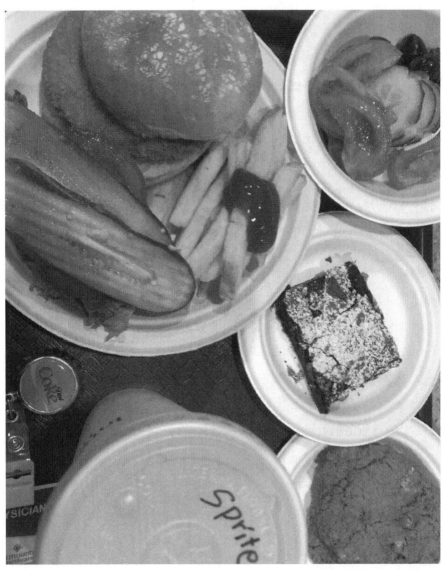

What in the world did people do in the old days without the hoard of prescription drugs that surround us today? You might ask how did humans even survive without drugs at all? The answer is simple. We didn't need them.

Example #1: white processed sugar was not loaded into everything from our breakfast eggs to your late evening so-called healthy yogurt, therefore diabetes drugs were not needed (because few if any actually had the disease to begin with).

Example # 2: attention deficit disorder in 19% of children in US--a hyperactivity disorder. Before toxic food colorings, MSG, processed sugar and hundreds of other hazardous chemicals were fed to children, destroying their gut bacteria while being disguised as food, there was no such thing as 'attention-deficit' and therefore no drugs were needed for children.

Example # 3: 800,000 people die each year with heart disease. Before inflammatory causing processed factory-made fake foods (hydrogenated trans fats) arrived on our shelves, people didn't have much heart disease, and therefore drugs for cholesterol, blood thinning and blood pressure were not needed.

Example # 4: Cancer. Hundreds if not thousands of sci-entific studies once again prove that sugar and inflammatory foods and additives are the number one cause of cancer. When cancer patients are taken off of these harmful chemicals, cancer cells die. Cancer cannot survive without inflammation and therefore no dangerous chemotherapy and radiation drugs were needed.

Example # 5: Alzheimer's. The Alzheimer's Association estimates that one in ten people over the age of sixty-five and nearly half of the folks over eighty-five years-old will eventually have the disease. Once again take a look at the turmeric studies at UCLA and other universities. They are not only preventing the disease but are now actually reversing it in some patients by stopping inflammation.

These are only a few examples, and I'm sure most of us over the age of fifty remember a time when most ninety year-olds could remember and share stories of their whole lives. They did not have what I call *the chemically-induced modern-day disease called Alzheimer's* or any form of foggy thinking.

Now let's talk about this cholesterol thing. Have you ever in your life heard so much chatter about this one thing? You can't even go to the gym or dinner and a movie with friends anymore without the topic of cholesterol coming up. I speak to people daily about their health and have met men and women in their twenties who have excellent health but their total cholesterol level starts to approach 200 and their doctors scare them to death and prescribe dangerous drugs--and this usually happens when their HDL and LDL levels are perfectly good! It's as if the medical Association works for the pharmaceutical companies, hmmm. Most of the doctors that are doing this don't even check to see if their patients have any inflammation markers. I have a sixty-five year-old friend who has been on cholesterol drugs for fifteen years. When I asked her if she actually had any blood lipid problems, her answer was no. Her doctor has given her drugs which are destroying her body for fifteen years simply because her mother had heart problems. Folks, that's nuts. That is the same as automatically putting an anti-leak fluid in your new engine just because your old car needed it.

Any doctor who abuses their patients to this degree should certainly lose their medical license. In my personal opinion this is not only malpractice, it is criminal. If we don't start opening our eyes to this pharmaceutical conspiracy, most of us are on a horrific path to destruction.

Below is an example of a handout given to a friend of mine from his doctor. It was meant to show some suggested healthy substitutions for commonly eaten sweets. Notice how inflammatory and very unhealthy all of these are. (Sugar-free is sweetened with artificial flavors and usually has MSG and other hidden dangerous chemicals added):

Sweets	
Eat	Sugar substitutes; sugar-free, low fat/fat free sweets & desserts; sugar-free gelatin; sugar-free pudding made with skim milk; fat-free fudgesicles with no added sugar, sugar-free popsicles
	Fat-free frozen yogurt; sherbet; sorbet; fat-free desserts; angel food cake; gingersnaps; marshmallows;
Don't Eat	White sugar; brown sugar; honey; jam; jelly; syrup; cake; pound cake; pie; cookies; ice cream; regular pudding; custard; chocolate; candy

If you are somewhat unsure of my wisdom, take a survey of someone you know--a parent, spouse, brother or sister or maybe even a friend who has been taking cholesterol medicine for longer than six months. Ask them if their health has improved with their medication, and what their doctor has prescribed to them for proper nutrition. I can tell you the answer before you ask. Here is how it goes down:

First your doctor prescribes you with a small 10 mg. dosage of cholesterol medication and tells you it won't hurt you, and in the same breath he tells you that you are in a state of pre-heart disease (not really a disease), and that you should only eat low-fat everything. He doesn't mention any advice about inflammation or sugar, and then he tells you to come back in six months, all while he is done with you and walking out the door. You then leave and walk to your car and look in the mirror looking like a deer in the headlights and stare, all the while wondering if you're going to make it home alive.

Next, you and your spouse hurry to your local mega giant fake food grocery store to purchase your so-called life-saving food--(first big mistake). You buy all of the low-fat foods you can find assuming that you will be healed soon and be able to get off of that dreaded cholesterol medication. Think again.

You just did two things horribly wrong that day. First you took the drugs that will wreak havoc on your health, and then you purchased processed foods (sugar) that have no life sustaining healthy saturated (not trans) fats. Then six to twelve months later you go back to your doctor and your blood lipid panel shows that your HDL good cholesterol is crashing downward to an unhealthy low (due simply from taking the healthy fats out of your diet). Your doctor then tells you that your health is getting worse and your blood tests show a widening ratio of total to HDL cholesterol. He then recommends bumping your drug dose from 10 mg up to 20 mg. Is this story starting to sound familiar, folks? Well you think he is the doctor, and once again you head straight back to the giant fake food store to shop for food with even less fat.

Now during this harmful process most of us don't even think or care about how much sugar, MSG or other inflammatory chemicals are on the ingredient list because your doctor never mentioned about anything but fat. Well folks, what I say to that is "FIRE YOUR DOCTOR". You don't work for him--he works for you! And if he's not helping you get well, let him go and find a better one. You wouldn't keep taking your car to a mechanic who couldn't fix it, so why would you take your body, your soul and your life to someone who can't or won't help you fix it?

As time passes and your good HDL cholesterol continues to stay down in the unhealthy range, this creates small blood particles that embed into your artery walls. These particles then build up into what is known as plaque, which in turn raises blood pressure. "Oh no," you say--this calls for even lower fat food because after all, isn't this what we and our doctors are being taught by big pharma? What a joke! That's like the fox teaching the chicken to leave the door of the henhouse unlocked at night! In the blink of an eye you went from being a healthy, awesome, beautiful person to some sickling on choles- terol and blood pressure medicine. Guess again!

You are sicker than you thought because your doctor then tells you with the hardening of your arteries, you absolutely without a doubt need to be taking a blood thinning drug or you will surely die from the heart problems, (all of which are more than likely caused by the three drugs your doctor prescribed to you in the first place)! So now you're thinking, my doctor caused all this? Yes, and this scenario happens more often than you could ever imagine.

If only your doctor had simply instructed you to start eating healthy fruits and veggies and saturated fats including wild caught fish, grass-fed beef, pork, chicken, real lard (¼ the saturated fat as butter) and other oils like olive and coconut oil, and raw grass-fed unpasteurized milk and butter, and to stay away from high fructose corn syrup and processed, chem- ical-laced fake so-called foods! The odds are very, very high that you would still be in excellent health and would never have had to take any medication to start with! Wow, you say, *I could have saved myself that easily, but now I'm surely doomed.* Okay, just calm down a little and take a deep breath because we all know that stress is surely another cause of disease. And actually, no, if you are still reading this book then you are alive and well and have an excellent chance to learn the truth and make the changes that will dramatically return your health back to excellence.

It's mind-boggling when every scientific study tells us something totally different from what really works. Just keep one thing in mind: scientists have to make a living just as we do and are funded nonstop by donations because they supposedly keep discovering new so-called facts. I say they are wrong and I can prove it. (When all of you obese sickly scientists get tired of watching yourselves and your own families suffer with disease, give me a call and let's talk).

The cat's been out of the bag for some time now and you and I both know that all of these new phony cholesterol guidelines (that have been made up by the pharmaceutical companies), suggesting very unhealthy total and LDL levels, are only for the benefit of selling more drugs. The new recommended LDL cholesterol level of 70 is not only impossible but totally unhealthy. The pharmaceutical companies are aware that almost all human beings cannot achieve a level of 70 by any means except malnutrition and medications which automatically put you in scare mode. There are also two kinds of LDL and most doctors conveniently forget to mention this fact. LDL can have large particles or small. High levels of LDL with large particles just happen to be perfectly healthy. The small particles are the ones that embed into your arteries and cause clots. Ask your doctor for this specific test before you take drugs. The negative effects of the cholesterol-lowering drugs are less than exciting--things like memory loss, permanent pain, gout, diabetes, cirrhosis, and damaged elevated liver enzymes. Why just what a person needs, right? And you most likely didn't even need to be doped up to begin with! Why in the heck didn't your doctor just tell you to go home and eat some beans? Well, your auto mechanic surely wouldn't tell you how to keep your car from ever breaking down would he?

And beans you ask? Yes, beans and ground flaxseed are some of the healthiest foods you can consume for cholesterol-lowering benefits. Your good 'ole doc didn't tell you that one did he? Beans and flaxseed also help to lower blood sugar and metabolize insulin levels. And remember, cholesterol doesn't cause clogged arteries, *inflammation* of cholesterol does.

Your body produces 75% of it's cholesterol through your liver and cells, and even more from the liver as your cells need it. Cholesterol is essential for building natural vitamin D, testosterone and estrogen. When a (dangerous) unnatural pharmaceutical medicine unnaturally lowers cholesterol and your vitamin D crashes as the direct result, then the immune system is lowered to dangerous levels that can no longer protect you from disease. Using cholesterol lowering drugs to mask something that may not even be a problem to start with and causing many more problems in the process--no that is not my idea of good healing.

Another suggestion to help lower your LDL cholesterol is

to consume a good dose of plant sterols. Be sure to get them from natural organic fruits and vegetables and not from supplements, because synthetic supplements just will not work like real whole foods. And don't even look at the liver-killing fake food products that are 'fortified' with artificial plant sterols. Once again, your new healthy lifestyle the John Rankin Way will consist of real foods to heal your body. You will certainly lose the battle if you are only slightly convinced by misleading marketing. So please, please, please stay with me folks while I explain these things in more detail. What do you have to lose? I'm assuming you have tried everything else and haven't been healed yet!

HEALED BY FARM
CHAPTER EIGHT

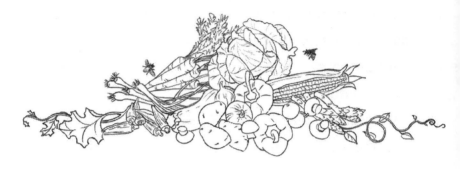

RAISING CHILDREN IN THE
MIDST OF THE FOOD CON ERA

"My teenage years were typical of most kids growing up in this country in the middle of the 20th century. Even though there was no visible sign of disease in my body, I was in a process that almost took my life years later."

Most of us remember what it's like being a teenager. We are either going to be one, have been one, are the parents of one, or are going to be the parents of one--God bless the latter. Teenage years are some of the most difficult in a person's life. As a parent, you observe your children changing from sweet innocent babies to raging hormone-driven monsters, by no fault of their own of course. They won't listen to good common sense, and all of a sudden they are much smarter than their parents. And worst of all is trying to feed a teenager. This has to be one of the most confusing things a parent will ever witness.

Just watch your kids in the morning as they are speeding out of the house at warp speed with wet hair and wrinkled clothes, grabbing all of the (so-called food) packages that you bought for them at the local mega fake food store. And by the way, have you ever noticed just how big the mega fake food stores' shopping carts are? They look like a twin bed on wheels! Oh, that's right, they sell those also at those stores. I'm personally guilty of buying everything from televisions to refrigerators from those kinds of stores, but I can absolutely guarantee you that this is not the place to be shopping for all-natural real food your teenagers or anyone else in your family need.

Have you ever wondered just how your teenager can grow like a weed (obviously hormones) while eating nothing but processed refined chemicals all day long? Just read the labels! Imagine what your kids would look and feel like if you fed them real natural grass-fed meats, fish, raw dairy, nuts and seeds, real grains and organic fruits and vegetables every single day of their lives! There probably are not many studies available but I would bet that obesity, attention deficit, and diabetes is almost nonexistent in teenagers who live on rural farms.

All that I'm teaching you is a no-brainer, folks. How many of us, including myself, have invested countless hours for a dozen years coaching or sitting on the sidelines trying to make our kids the greatest athletes ever and then celebrate their big ballgame win by driving them straight to a fast-food restaurant? That little 'reward' is giving your child a lethal dose of trans fats, nitrates, genetically modified potassium bromate doused and bleached bread with enough carbohydrates, sugar, MSG, sodium, and other chemicals to put your child's health on the road to misery!

Again, no fault as a parent. We simply have been conned by very greed-driven people who are not concerned about your good health. Now is the time to stand up to the ruthless marketing that has been ruining our loved-ones health for decades. Folks, at this time in history our teenagers will not escape illness if all that goes into their body is processed sugars and chemicals. Parents in the last generation had enough trouble watching over our health as teenagers, but parents today have a whole new battle to fight. The fast-food industry and soda companies seem to have taken our nation's school lunch system hostage with dangerous junk food and sodas being the only food choices for our children to purchase. You surely don't think they donate those high school ball field scoreboards without an agenda do you?

I actually had someone in the medical profession tell me recently that a little bit of processed sugar is good for you! Of course my response was full of laughter because I absolutely know better. I often watch the constant flow of obese children walking the sidewalk at the school near my home. I dare any-one to tell those (pre-diabetic) kids that just a little bit of sugar won't hurt them! I'll step out on a limb here and bet that most parents have, on at least one or more occasions, protested to your child's coach to let your child play or bat first. But how many of us have ever once attended a school board meeting to protest the fact that the school lunch options are poisoning our precious children?

As parents, now is the time to step up to the plate and be vocal about the horrific nutrition scams that are promoted by mega giant fake food companies for the sole purpose of addict-ing your children and pleasing stockholders. And when shop-ping at the mega giant fake food store, it would be a good idea to only choose things like paper plates and batteries, but don't be fooled by the fake foods offered there. You certainly will not find anything except unhealthy feedlot animal products in the meat department. Like I said before, these are those animals fed a diet that consists mainly of genetically modified corn, soy-beans, antibiotics, growth hormones, and starchy by-products such as white bread and candy, certainly not a healthy choice for your children or yourselves.

And for your further education, know that these mega feed-lot cattle producers have gotten in on the truth about grass-fed meat and are trying to beat out the real grass-fed (mom and pop local farm) producers by coming up with some 'legal' governmental regulations to fool you again. As you probably have noticed lately, grass-fed labels are showing up on products in the mega stores more and more. BUYER BEWARE! Yes, in 2014, our trusty old feedlot giants talked their federal regulator buddies into passing a new law that allows beef to be labeled grass-fed if it is on pasture for three months out of the year. Notice I didn't say grass, just pasture. So in reality a cow can eat hay in January, February and March and then be fed genetically modified corn the next nine months of the year and still be sold as healthy grass-fed meat in our grocery stores (without that animal ever having eaten even a single blade of fresh grass). They are also feeding cattle compressed pellets of GMO corn and soybeans with a small amount of dry hay in it and (by law) can call it grass-fed! Wow, to consumers like you and I who are trying our best to be extremely healthy, that is very scary news. The reason we want grass-fed in the first place is because the fresh grass-fed animals are filled with life-saving ingredients that we want and need such as beta-carotene, CLA's (cancer-killers), vitamin D, calcium, and natural iodine, just to name a few--and you simply can't trust a fake grass-fed product to do that for you. This is just one great big

John Rankin

reason I warn folks to beware of their food supply sources. You just have no idea how far this con goes. Nothing mass-produced is the same as that bought from a naturally raised real food source--not even close. This food con madness should be a very big concern to every red-blooded American citizen.

My teenage years were typical of most kids growing up in this country in the middle of the 20th century. Even though there was no visible sign of disease in my body, I surely was in the process of something that almost took my life years later. During my youth, my daily intake of candy, soda, chips, and fast foods did however send me to the dentist quite regularly and give me constant stomach aches. And no, I wasn't gluten intolerant, (just like most of you are not). I had little or no healthy gut flora from the effects of all the junk I ate plus all the antibiotics I took for my root canals. (Just like you?)

I talk to people about their health on a daily basis and I often hear the same comments: "I eat all of the junk food trash I want and it hasn't hurt me yet." Or they might say, "You have to die sometime." To such completely irresponsible and ignorant comments I will just say this: "Our Creator has given us a most unique and wonderful earth to sustain our lives while we are here--for a reason. It's all been designed perfectly to sustain a very good (healthy) life for every one of God's children. So please always remember to never mock these gifts or to take them for granted. Show your gratitude by learning all you can and making wise choices--and don't be conned".

My wife and I recently got a good dose of how the marketing schemes from the mega fake food companies are preying on our children and ultimately destroying their lives. We attended our five-year-old grandson's 'Grandparent's Day Luncheon' at his preschool. Besides the fact that the food was not really something fit for human consumption, we made the best of it and still really enjoyed being with our beautiful grand-son. When lunch was over we did the typical meet-the-teacher thing. Then I noticed a few racks of books for sale and some-one standing next to them at a cash register. I was informed by my five-year-old grandson that it was 'Book Fair Day' and each child could purchase a book to take home. Without hesitation I reached into my pocket and pulled out money for him to pur-chase a book. But when I saw the books available to the kids, I instantly became very protective of my grandson as though

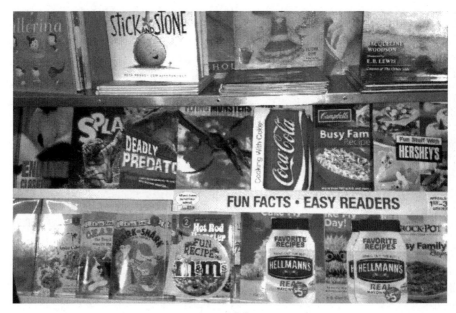

a predator was about to attack him! I was absolutely shocked by the incredible presentation of propaganda in his book choices! (See the photo here that I took of those book choices). Fortunately he chose a good book and was not impressed by the attempted con. I am very serious when I say food companies are without conscious in preying on our young children for purposes of promoting the fake food lie and addicting children for financial gain.

As we exited the school we decided to go to a new children's movie at the local theater. The movie seemed innocent enough but when it was over, I had counted dozens of times throughout the movie that an animated car was fueled with three kinds of slurpees, candy, sodas and chips--all as part of the movie theme.

If he hadn't been marketed to enough by what I had already seen at his school and at the theater, as we returned to my grandson's home I noticed him playing with a toy that had a sugar-cereal advertisement on it! After a day like that, what do you think my five-year-old grandson would be thinking about? Well you can guess what the deceiving marketing teams of those fake food companies would like for him to be thinking about...and it's anything but about being healthy!

Although my daughter prepares wholesome delicious real food daily for my grandson, this kind of shameful propaganda thrown at small children everywhere we look makes it an uphill battle for parents to keep their children healthy. Once again--do the math folks.

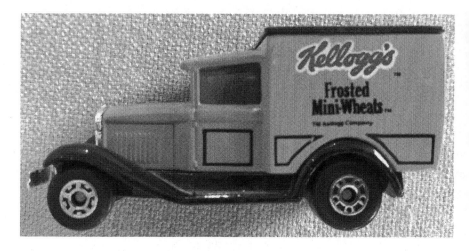

HEALED BY FARM
CHAPTER NINE

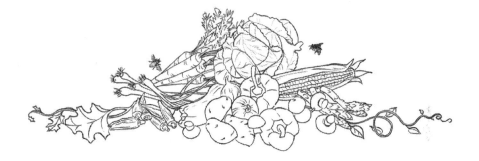

MY SECOND DOSE OF REALITY

*"Could my mother or yours have been or still be
saved from tragic death with the understanding
that we now have?"*

As if my teenage years were not hard enough, I was soon going to learn my hardest lesson of life. When I was twenty years old, my mother found out that she had non-Hodgkin's lymphoma. Needless to say, at such a young age I was in denial that anything could ever hurt my mother. Isn't this the way most of us feel when a family member or close friend first contacts a life-threatening disease? We always think that our mom or dad will just somehow miraculously get well, or that modern-day medicine will cure them. Think again.

For the next seven years, while so-called 'modern' medicine invaded her once beautiful body, I sat and held my mother's hand and watched her slowly die a horrific death. During those seven years, my mother and I worked closely together doing the best we knew at the time, creating new juice and food concoctions we hoped would kill her cancer. The things my mother and I learned certainly extended her suffering for about five years longer than her doctors expected.

Watching my mother lose her hair and become extremely sick from chemotherapy drugs (over and over for seven years) only angered me, because I had great faith and trust that the doctors and all of the glorious new drugs would certainly heal her. It is devastating for a son at age twenty-seven to watch his mother take her last breath while holding her hand.

I have riddled myself with guilt for many years since then because I was helpless and deprived of the knowledge and understanding to keep my mother alive and healthy. Fortunately that life-saving information now exists. Actually it always did, I just didn't know it in time to use it to save my mother's life. The unfortunate fact is that modern-day scientific research is paid for by mega-food companies and drug companies. This is the reason my mother's body could not heal naturally and rid itself of the cancer, and why thirty-four years later still no cure exists.

I watched her eat numerous bowls of processed ice cream and other sugary desserts, all while the cancer cells (free radicals) ate away at her internal organs. Since the day of her death all those years ago, nothing has changed in the world of unethical and inexcusable marketing. Every doctor, magazine advertisement, or television commercial assured my mother that eating everything from margarine, sugar, food dyes, monosodium glutamate, to inflammatory hydrogenated cooking oils was the new healthy and modern way of preparing food. The refined-food marketers also convinced my mother through (purely evil in my opinion) misleading science that the very things Mother Nature put here--lard, real butter, raw dairy, and grass fed meat--were actually harmful to her body. SHAME ON THEM.

You may ask the question, why would the food companies conspire against us in this way? If you have to ask, I have just one answer: PROFIT!!! I will repeat myself on this issue and assure you that a food processor's first goal is to consistently increase profit margins for their shareholders. Helping you get and stay healthy is never on their list of things to consider for their job description, only making you think your health is their concern is a priority--part of the con.

The things I've learned through my life full of many such 'wake up calls' caused me to decide that I had to know the truth about health. I will share more of these life-changing experiences throughout this book, but know that because of this and other such reality checks, I chose to make myself what you might call a human guinea pig. I have spent years practicing every kind of natural remedy on myself, hoping to avoid suffering an untimely death like so many of my loved-ones.

I have learned that such things as processed hydrogenated cooking oils and margarine (derived from man-made synthetic dangerous chemicals) do not even come close to replicating the natural healing powers that our Creator put on earth with natural foods meant to sustain a healthy lifestyle. This is not just my radical theory. Studying the history of health in the American people proves my case, as history absolutely leaves a clear and vivid trail of this truth. To support my theory, note that the onslaught of diseases like childhood leukemia, heart disease, cancer, Alzheimer's, diabetes, Crohn's disease, anxiety, multiple sclerosis, thyroid disease, Parkinson's, ADHD and autism and many other autoimmune diseases--just to name a few pieces of evidence--found their way into our society immediately following the commercialization of the food industry--creating many forms of what I call 'imitation' or fake food.

As I have mentioned so many times, nearly all disease starts in the body from an inflammatory response. These responses are almost always centered on gut bacteria, also known as microflora--the bacteria that eat what we eat. If you have a concern for your health or have a disease such as heart disease, cancer, or particularly irritable bowel syndrome, you need to pay particular attention to your gut bacteria. The latest studies prove the old saying, you are what you eat. This is a big one I wish I had known when my mother was suffering the cancer. I'm quite sure we could have beat it if we had only known.

The human body actually has two nervous systems. The one that most of us are familiar with is the central nervous system which consists of our brain and spinal cord. Most of us have been taught that the central nervous system in the brain is responsible for making most of the decisions in our body. WRONG. The less spoken about but very powerful and more influential nervous system is the colon. A recently discovered nerve named the vagus nerve extends from the colon to the brain. Another recent discovery is that our colon sends much more information through this nerve than the brain sends. In other words, the 37 trillion cells in our body are controlled by our 100 trillion gut bacteria. All of this seems very complicated but really it's quite simple: **whether or not we have a pure healthy functioning body and mind is the result of our personal food choices in daily life.**

Here is how it works: good healthy gut bacteria are killed

by things like antibiotics, store-bought bread additives (like bleach and potassium bromate), and many other chemicals used in our food supply. Then the gut sends a message to the brain that the good bacteria are dead. The brain in response sends out an alarm to the organs that there are not enough anti-inflammatories and the body is in trouble. Without correcting the gut bacteria by ingesting healthy nutrients such as real probiotics and natural anti-inflammatories, the free radicals (inflammation) become rampant and disease starts in the body. Just know that the alarm is always sounding if you are eating fake food, so you must consciously choose to eat only anti-inflammatory real food regularly.

Use your common sense folks and take care of your health. It is very easy to prevent or fix this situation. First, eat probiotics and other healthy bacteria. My recommendation is to get these from fermented vegetables, raw unpasteurized milk, yogurt, butter and cheese from grass-fed cows, goats or sheep. I do not recommend getting it from a bottle of pasteurized chemicals found on the grocery store shelves. I also do not recommend getting it from a bottle of pills from a synthetic food processor.

Your good gut bacteria are reinstated back into your body immediately after taking in some healthy probiotics. But then it is vital that you change your food intake to include only anti-inflammatory foods. Almost all states allow raw grass-fed dairy to be sold. A good website to help you locate local sources is *www.realmilkfinder.com.*

A daily intake of omega-3 fatty acids will help reduce inflammation to undetectable levels in your body. These can be sourced with such foods as salmon, tuna, eggs, nuts, plants, and flaxseed. Another concern is our daily balance between omega-6 and omega-3. The balance is recommended at a one-to-one ratio, but in the Western civilization that ratio is often unbalanced to as much as 30 to 1 ratio. This happens as a consequence of eating hydrogenated oils in most processed and fast food. This unbalanced 30 to 1 ratio is very dangerous and causes a human body to become very acidic and inflammatory, creating an environment friendly to all diseases.

To enjoy perfect health, I eat only pure raw unpasteurized dairy and extra-virgin oils such as lard, coconut oil, and olive oil from very reliable sources. I eat fresh organic fruits, vegetables, garlic, nuts and seeds and whole grains every day. "Yes, I did say the so-called and often-denoted bad word *grain* which I'll explain later in the book". I will also support my claims later in this book by sharing how my personal health changed from bad to great, including success stories of others as well who are living the same John Rankin's Way lifestyle and eating the same real foods.

Could my mother or yours have been or still be saved from tragic death with the understanding that we now have about what our Creator's true intention is for the foods offered for the good health of his children? I would say absolutely and without hesitation, yes!

HEALED BY FARM
CHAPTER TEN

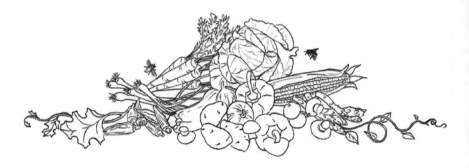

MY TIME TO GROW UP

"None of our genepool had any disease whatsoever before the mega giant (fake) food companies corrupted our food. I personally proved them wrong, and that it had absolutely nothing to do with genetics."

Losing a loved one when you are young will certainly help you grow up fast, whether you want to or not. I spent seven long years observing the workings of the hospital and was not the least bit enthused with what I had learned. From the smells, sounds, and sight of every intravenous machine known to mankind, I determined to never return there once we had buried my dear mother. There is just one small thing I have failed to mention--well, it seems small compared to chemotherapy.

Three years into my mother's cancer, my father had open-heart surgery. It seemed as though he made it through this, with the exception of having to take a few prescription drugs daily. Therein lies the problem in those two little words: prescription drugs. How many of us either consume or watch someone consume the little wonders of the pharma-ceutical industry only to watch their health continue on a downward spiral?

Taking the health-care advice of the medical profession and the American Heart Association, the state of my father's health continued to decline. IMAGINE THAT. Most physician's favorite response when they don't know how to heal someone is to blame it on genetics, and we have to just accept it. Yes, that's what they told my father. I say baloney. I was told those very same words by every doctor and nurse in the hospital. Is this what they teach every nurse to say to their patients? "Oh well, you can't do anything about it, it's genetics". Funny how none of our genepool had any disease whatsoever before the mega giant food companies corrupted our food. I personally proved them wrong, and in my case also proved it had absolutely nothing to do with genetics. That's another story that I will discuss later on in the book.

So just what did the AHA recommend that further damaged my father's health? (They are supposed to be the good guys, right?) I've since discovered it depends on who the big donations come from as to whose good guys they are. One of the things you would never think you have to battle is our very own heart association and cancer society, right? The next time you sit down in a restaurant and order a meal with a heart healthy logo beside it, just be aware that the food is more than likely loaded with disease-causing inflammatory things that you do not want to put in your body. As I have mentioned earlier, restaurant chains (not you) donate millions of dollars to these so-called nonprofit groups. For those of you who frequently eat out at restaurants (especially fast food) you need to be very aware of what is on the menu and just where the food originated. Did it come from somewhere such as China, where they have a record of growing and processing contaminated food?

Some of you may be asking me the question, "So then we can never go out for dinner and enjoy ourselves again?" My answer is yes and no. No you should not eat what kills you, and yes you will enjoy yourselves much more than you have ever imagined if you don't eat out at unhealthy restaurants. Find ways to always eat only real natural foods.

We have touched on things such as hydrogenated oils and sugar, but most of us don't have any idea of the harm being done by the very deceptive and common overuse of monosodium glutamate (MSG). This poison has been around much longer than most of us have. We started hearing about it in the late 1970's and early 80's when the talk about it as a Chinese food additive was spreading around the country (about as fast as the addition of many new restaurants using it). Those of us who were fairly health-conscious knew enough to simply ask our waiters to leave it out of our meal. Odds are that your message never made it to the kitchen...and it probably wouldn't have made much of a difference anyway because all of the meats, rice, soy and egg rolls come from giant (unethical) fake food companies and are already pumped full of MSG as a flavor enhancer in order to make cheap unhealthy processed foods taste delicious. You don't honestly think for one minute that the all-you-can-eat $4.95 special is actually from ingredients other than diseased feedlots or cheap contaminated producers do you? C'mon folks, quit fooling yourselves.

MSG was invented by a Japanese chemist named Kikunae Ikeda in 1908. His sole purpose in isolating this chemical was to make an artificial seaweed flavor as a food additive. (Word of caution: anytime we read the word additive on the ingredients list, run away quickly). MSG was not much of a problem in America for the first half of the 20th century. But during WWII, American soldiers capturing Japanese soldiers noticed that the Japanese food rations were much tastier than the US food rations. Yes, those Japanese rations were loaded with MSG.

It was in 1959 that the FDA ruled without any known studies (imagine that) that MSG was safe to be consumed by Americans. It would take five chapters to fully explain the science of MSG, but the bottom line is that it is made from glutamic acid, an excitotoxin which puts all 37 trillion of your cells on extreme overload (inflammation) causing cell death. (Just so you know, things like paint thinner are excitotoxins--is this what you want in your food source)? Scientific studies prove that these chemicals cause everything from obesity to Alzheimer's disease. Here's a little known fact: scientists studying obesity actually inject animals solely with MSG to intentionally fatten them in order to conduct their studies on obesity.

The sad part in all of this is the true fact that food refineries not only add this deadly substance to 99.9% of all processed foods but go as far as to disguise it under another food name or the often used *natural flavor* name--legally! As I've mentioned before, if it's safe for Americans to consume then why do food producers spend hundreds of millions of dollars lobbying politicians to hide it from us? Have you ever noticed after finishing a Chinese meal from a restaurant or any other restaurant that uses it, that as you're traveling home you look in your rearview mirror only to see a red swollen tingling face with inflamed hands and a slight headache, not to mention a really strong aftertaste that doesn't go away for days? The answer is yes, and our initial response is that we have just eaten too much. THINK AGAIN. I can certainly guarantee that you can overeat a healthy organic meal of grass-fed meat and non-pesticide fruits and vegetables and you will not have such a reaction, because overeating is not the problem! Eating Mother Nature's foods, you will actually prevent your body from inflaming and expanding like a balloon. Your liver and pancreas naturally work together with your colon to metabolize your insulin levels. By taking MSG out of your diet, you will not be exhausted and you will not feel like taking a nap after every meal--quite the opposite, you will feel and look like that awesome person you once were and or always wanted to be.

While we are on the topic of restaurant food, let's take a look at some of the other products we eat there that not only make us fatter and fatter but are causing disease in our bodies. This is another witness to what I like to refer to as *the con game*. The mega fake food companies are conning us as innocent consumers and playing a game with our family's health. We have been conned into thinking that foods labeled "50% less fat" or the word 'light' are healthier for us. Those words actually translate to the very fact that if you eat them, you will ultimately lose the battle of the bulge--and here's why. When you eat at a restaurant and order the (imaginary) low-fat salad with grilled chicken and light balsamic vinegar, here's what you actually get: the chicken that you're consuming has been brought from birth to maturity and then to slaughter in six weeks, fed a genetically modified corn and soybean (sugar) diet with growth hormones and heavy amounts of antibiotics. By comparison a healthy farm raised chicken grows to an adult in sixteen weeks. Next, these six-week-old mass-produced unhealthy chickens are taken to a factory and injected with monosodium glutamate, refined sodium, sugar, and washed with bleach, just to mention a few of the additives. Some are also processed so much they are soft as lunch meat or hard as a rock. Yum?

Then, of course, while you are waiting for the chef to grill your already chemicalized chicken, you are picturing it cooking and being glazed with a natural healthy oil and unrefined herbs and spices direct from the garden...yeah right! What really is happening in the kitchen is the chef is drowning your chicken with a butter-colored, inflammatory, low-grade genetically modified corn and/or soybean oil with another round of monosodium glutamate, refined sodium, and yes, sugar added from their so-called seasoning.

As the waiter sits the (gallon-size) grilled chicken salad in front of us, everyone at the table will usually request a 'light' salad dressing because it's healthier and it will help us lose weight. NOPE. And here's where it gets tricky. As we dump the balsamic vinegar over our salad we just assume it's healthy because, after all, it's balsamic vinegar. But real balsamic vinegar is made from fine Italian Trebbiano grapes that are aged, pressed, and fermented. Real balsamic vinegar is aged in wooden barrels from ten to one-hundred years and costs $30-$500 or more per bottle. So don't think for one second the fake stuff you're about to put on your salad that comes in a $3.95 bottle is anything but the following: water, genetically modified corn or soybean oil, canola, vegetable oils, vinegar, artificial coloring, low-grade olive oil, sugar, MSG, and very heavy doses of refined inflammatory sodium. All of these ingredients are highly inflammatory and will make your body fat and not thin as you had supposed. But, of course, we are eating this salad to lose weight, right? We would like to think so, but unfortunately again we have been duped by the food industry. And why you ask? The answer is the same as always: it's cheap to manufacture and very addictive.

Now let's take a real look into what was actually in the salad that we thought would help us to lose weight. First of all, if the fats in the oils were of pure natural lard, olive oil, coconut oil or grass-fed butter, then you would actually burn bad fat from your body and nourish yourself with extreme nutrition. But what you actually got from that restaurant salad is extreme oxidation, insulin imbalance, and inflammation from highly refined hydrogenated oils and chemicals, MSG and refined sodium--all of which adds weight to your body and feeds the growth of cancer cells, heart disease, diabetes, and Alzheimer's. All of this is horrible enough without the factory bread and restaurant low grade olive oil (which is usually diluted with canola oil from the supplier). Please tell me you don't eat this kind of food!

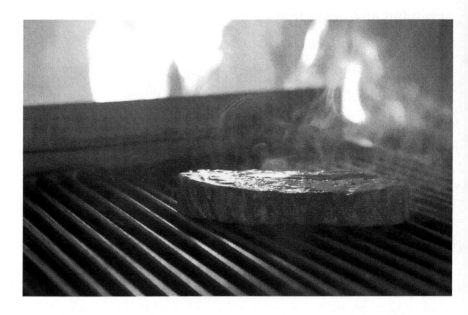

I may seem to be giving sodium a bad rap throughout the book, but let me explain: not all sodium is created equal, just like all food is not equal. Doctors are half right when they suggest salt will raise your blood pressure. Unfortunately, what most doctors don't understand is the simple fact that there is a product we can call inflammatory refined sodium and another product called anti-inflammatory unrefined sodium. If only this one small simple ingredient alone was taught in medical school and translated to patients, many heart attacks and cancer cases could be prevented. Funny how wild animals are not running around the earth with constant high blood pressure from eating salt out of the ground like they naturally do.

Of course theirs is non-refined. Most Americans have spent their entire lives consuming not only the same name brand of salt but also being totally unaware of how it is mined and processed. Most people just assume our everyday table salt is mined and then fine ground and ready for the table. THINK AGAIN.

Most refined sodium is cooked at over 1000° which oxidizes it and instantly makes it inflammatory to the human body. It is then bleached and mixed with a good dose of aluminum powder as an anti-caking agent--a very dangerous and toxic heavy metal that is known to be lethal to humans. Synthetic iodine is added to the list of ingredients, and then the one that always raises eyebrows--dextrose (sugar). Iodine imbalance is a big cause of goiter, thyroid dysfunction and mental retardation in children, so naturally we have all been taught to use only iodized salt to be sure we get the necessary Iodine in our bodies. If this is true then just how in the world did humans even survive all these thousands of years before the salt refineries came to our rescue?

Consider that these refineries heat the salt to oblivion, killing any naturally existing iodine. Then they conveniently come to our rescue by adding the substance they took out in the first place--but the problem is, they add back a synthetic version. Salt naturally comes out of this beautiful earth with 84 trace minerals, enzymes, and electrolytes, including an abundant source of natural iodine. Refined sodium has a total of four minerals left over by the time it gets to your table, kind of in line with the rest of processed foods.

The simple solution is a salt in its real unadulterated natural form. The two most popular are pink Himalayan or Celtic sea salt. The Pink Himalayan is my favorite. These are real salts that are just mined, broken up and sent to your table with all 84 minerals still in them available to be easily absorbed by your body. Real natural salt was actually traded as a highly valued commodity by settlers when they first came to America. It was not put here on earth to sicken and kill us as modern medical history tries to prove. It did no such thing for thousands of

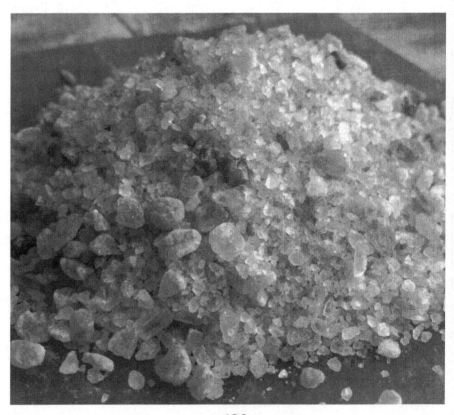

years until it was refined. Before I got on my present healthy diet, my body needed a magnesium and iodine supplement daily. But now I do not need that supplement because of the abundance of it in the all-natural unrefined sodium I use on my foods.

The test pictured below was done by pouring human urine over two grassy areas to test whether it had any effect on the healthy life of the plant. The plant on the right was doused two times daily for approximately five days from a human who was consuming refined inflammatory sodium as part of their regular diet. The plant on the left was doused three to four times daily for seventy-seven consecutive days from the same human who switched to all-natural pink Himalayan salt.

Plant life is naturally full of substances called polyphenols to protect themselves from things like disease and bugs, which

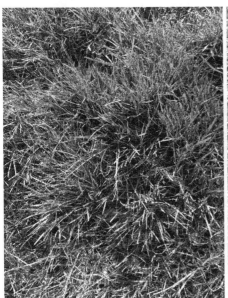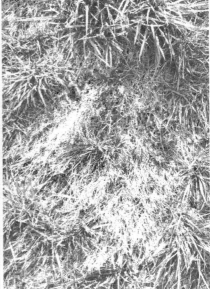

is the same polyphenol antioxidant supplied in fresh fruits and vegetables meant to help our bodies fight free radicals. It pretty much comes down to choosing which picture you would like your internal organs to look like. It's simple: the polyphenols in the plant on the right were 100% unable to protect the grass from the urine which included refined inflammatory salt, therefore it died. The same polyphenols in the grass on the left kept that grass from being destroyed by the urine which included unrefined healthy salt. That grass was not only protected but looked somewhat greener, probably because it was fertilized from the 84 minerals in the healthy salt! Pink Himalayan salt is probably the most alkalizing food on the face of the earth.

The final analysis of my 'salt in urine' research is that real unrefined sodium doesn't kill anything as suggested by most doctors, but instead it nourishes our bodies with wonderful nutrition. (And yes, this research was done by yours truly! And just know that the research also included a perfectly balanced real foods diet, not a junk food diet with some good salt added.)

Another very rich source of iodine is from consuming raw unpasteurized dairy. So for all of you folks with dysfunctional thyroids who are looking for a way to heal, you might want to try changing your salt and dairy before living (or dying) dependant on prescription drugs.

HEALED BY FARM
CHAPTER ELEVEN

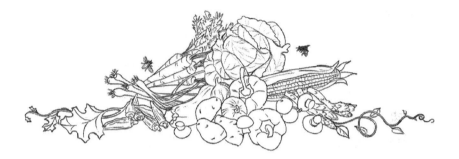

MIDDLE AGE BULGE

"As the inflammation leaves the body, so does the disease--it's that simple folks. It all comes down to this one thing: inflammation."

It happens to all of us. Sometime around the age of thirty, you're making a little money and can afford more nice things like eating out often with the kids...aah, the good life. And somewhere in that period of life, interestingly enough, another thing starts happening: your waist seems to thicken and soon it grows substantially larger. Your pant size, your shirt size, your health in general changes overnight before you know it.

As the old saying goes, been there done that. It happened to me too. Life experience is a great teacher. I'm here to tell you that we not only need to open our eyes, but also our hearts and minds and seek the truth about health. The problem is that when most of us are in our thirties, we have young children taking up most of our time and resources and maybe even making it difficult just to manage a normal day, (if you can ever call life normal with young children).

We are so engulfed in our children, their activities, and our careers at this time in our lives, we never slow down long enough to take a look in the mirror to see what's happening to our own personal health. What most of us see by the time we reach our thirties is that our skinny teenage bodies have filled out with fat bulges hanging out everywhere. All of a sudden when we think we have finally arrived at the peak of success we notice the changes, but perhaps we accept it because we look like most other adults.

It's anything but normal for an adult human body to expand it's size! By this time in life, some are probably earning enough to wine and dine at restaurants almost daily, and do! Another thing that most of us start to witness at this stage in our lives are the illnesses--and even deaths--of our loved-ones. I have personally experienced this exact life, and you will too if you haven't already, and especially if you eat the all-American diet.

But I have now found my even-healthier skinny teenage body once again simply by doing the things that I teach in this book. I get compliments all the time about my fitness and appearance. A large percentage of overweight people have diseased or pre-diseased bodies and horrific blood lipid panels and are totally unaware of it. What most of us don't understand is there is good news here: the very true exciting fact that as we change our diet to the way I teach as the John Rankin Way, our bodies will start shedding fat easily! Blood lipid panels such as cholesterol, thyroid, PSA, and C-reactive protein (inflammation marker) will return to a normal healthy young person's level. As the inflammation leaves the body, so does the disease--it's that simple folks. It all comes down to this one thing: inflammation.

Everywhere we look there are marketing ads (cons) trying to convince us that they have the absolute best 100% sure way to lose weight. They all sound wonderful (and will only cost about twice as much as just simply shopping for natural foods)! So why would we be willing to spend more for the new diet plan that your favorite movie star endorses?

It's simple. First, we let the television and magazine ads

market (con) us with wonderful promises that are not sustainable and actually do not work. Secondly, we all want something that absolutely cannot happen in the human body: the quick and easy fix. Oh yes, if just one of these marketing 'scams' worked at all, then why is it that almost every single person we are acquainted with in our daily lives is still trying to lose weight year after year after year? Some of the major weight-loss companies even have monthly meetings where the participants meet and talk about their weight loss problems. These meetings amount to nothing more than people shedding their emotions and having a rah-rah party. I don't know about you folks, but when I have a problem of any sort in life, I usually don't go and talk with a couple dozen other folks who have the same problem as I do. I seek out someone who has actually fixed that problem, and I would hope you would do the same!

US Obesity Levels 1990-2016

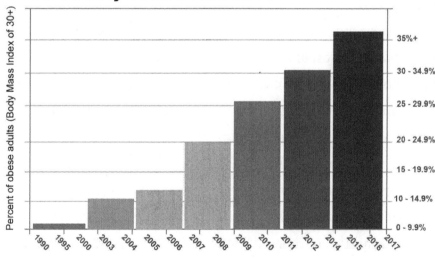

Source: Trust for America's Health and Robert Wood Johnson Foundation, "The State of Obesity," stateofobesity.org, Sep. 2016

Another form of misleading marketing is through the use of fitness models and bodybuilders. Everyone wants to look like these guys, right? So naturally we want to consume the same protein powders, bars, snacks, and weight loss supplements that they do. WRONG AGAIN! The only problem is that after eating these products and spending our hard-earned cash, we still don't look like them. And guess what: the models don't actually look the way they do by eating those hydrogenated oxidized inflammatory poisons either. Now don't let this burst your bubble, because anyone can get in great shape with enough education, discipline, and by following a little common sense--which I teach. In reality, most of these magazine models are very young, have naturally lean bodies, and just haven't been exposed to enough years of bodily abuse to be fat yet. Their diet usually consists of *light* everything, eliminating healthy thyroid. muscle and hormone building saturated fats completely.

A fitness model/ bodybuilder can be conned also. They have been taught that real foods with real healthy fats will make their bodies fat, which is absolutely not true. Real healthy foods including healthy fats do not make you fat. Two weeks prior to a fitness competition, these guys start a 'starvation period' which is basically total malnutrition. We only assume by their looks that they are very healthy. Wrong again--the total opposite is true. The starvation is the reason that they get very lean and all of their ribs start to show. This is common knowledge. Now just take one guess when the pictures for these magazine ads are taken of the bodybuilders and fitness models--yes, during the starvation period. These are danger- ous choices and dangerous supplements being sold by these models. Talk about not seeing the forest for the trees! I have absolutely proven that eating healthy the John Rankin Way creates a lean body with gorgeous muscles built from regular normal workouts.

Although I do come down hard on misleading products, their manufacturers, and endorsers, I do acknowledge that I'm an avid fan of the gym and physical exercise. I guess besides the strong addictive physical benefit of working out regularly for nearly forty years, the fact is that exercise greatly reduces cortisol, the stress hormone. I often hear the phrase, "as soon as I get the stress off of me I'm going to start working out", and of course I immediately answer with a frown. That's kind of like the chicken or the egg story, which came first.

I don't speak much about exercise in this book but let me just say this much: do it often. Regardless of what age you are now, combining exercise with eating real foods will change your life back to the strong healthy person you once were in your youth. I speak to men and women every day about their weight, and most of them are under the impression that they can just do more cardio and the pounds will come off--again not true. Let me make it very clear that it is physically impos- sible to outwork a bad diet at the gym. When you are eating a

diet high in carbohydrates, processed sugars, and hydrogenated oils, and doing exhausting cardio workouts, your body just
craves more fuel. Here's where the slope gets slippery. Unfortunately, the kind of fuel your body craves is more of the addictive fake food you have been eating in order to satisfy your
out-of-control insulin spikes. So you did burn a few calories,
but afterwards you feed your liver and pancreas much more of
the inflammatory, weight-gaining ingredients than you were
eating in the first place. It's obviously a losing battle and simply will not and has not ever worked for weight management.

This whole weight-loss marketing scam has it all totally
wrong, selling us the lie that it's all about calories and low-
fat. If this were even remotely true, then how in the world
would our ancestors have been so healthy and lean? They
never counted a single calorie, nor did they know what one
was! They ate plenty of calories from their homegrown vegetables and fruits, grains, and nuts, and their diet consisted of
naturally produced oils, meats, fish, eggs, and dairy fats. Can
you just imagine that your very lean great-great-grandmother
was sitting around her cabin worrying about how many calories
she was consuming? When you eat natural foods, your body
will tell you when to quit eating and your hunger will subside
for hours.

The most common quote I hear everyday is, "Well John,
people worked really hard back in the old days and that's how
they stayed lean". I have spent the biggest part of my life work-

ing around construction workers who do hard physical labor ten to twelve-hours daily in the hot sun and they are anything but lean. The difference of course is that the construction workers snack on doughnuts and potato chips and wash it down with a soft drink all day long. Your ancestors snacked on wild berries, raw carrots, and tomatoes while working all day long.

When I was in my mid-thirties, I grew from my high school weight of 165 pounds to what I thought was a healthy 214 pounds. I grew from a 30-inch to a 36-inch waist, and from a medium shirt to an extra-large. At thirty-five years old I was 21% body fat. As a 6'3" tall teen I was very self-conscious about being too skinny. So I simply did what many young men did: to gain weight I ate everything in sight (including inflammatory hydrogenated trans fats and sugars). The only problem was that those eating habits almost ended my life a few decades later.

So I have news for all of you high school football players who want to get big. BE AWARE! Looking back to my thirties, I was fairly satisfied with my larger size except for one little thing that I just couldn't get rid of, no matter how hard I exercised--the love handles (or as I like to refer to them now--the inflammation handles)! I engaged in doing countless ab and cardio classes at the gym just to see my belly fat grow. I tried every supplement and everything modern-day science teaches us, only to have worse results.

After changing my diet to what I teach in the John Rankin's Way, my body weight is now 194 pounds. My waist is 32 inches. I wear a medium to large shirt once again. And I am very healthy at 11½% body fat. This size is back to what I was when I was twenty years old, not to mention my extremely healthy blood panel is worthy of some serious coveting. And guess what--I once again eat everything in sight! But it just happens that every morsel of food that is in my kitchen and that goes into my mouth is from an all-natural, unrefined (uncorrupted), and disease-preventing real food source.

At 6'3", I never thought I would feel comfortable dropping my weight back below two hundred pounds. With my height (as most men feel) I had always assumed I would look more manly weighing over two hundred pounds. But what I have learned is that it is extremely more manly to be sixty years old and as healthy as a ten year old. There's absolutely nothing manly about being inflamed, sick, and overweight and unnecessarily sticking needles into your gut twice a day like all of you diabetics have to do to manage your insulin levels, all while not being able to even urinate like a normal man.

With my transition back to great health, I have also started to experience better vision, improved cognitive skills, less body fat, higher energy and hormone levels, and much more muscle mass. As self-conscious as I once was in my younger years about being too thin, now when a friend or acquaintance calls me skinny I just smile and ask them if they are interested in achieving the same results. Unfortunately Americans have been programmed into believing that increased body fat with age is natural, acceptable, and normal. I'm here to tell you it's anything but that.

HEALED BY FARM
CHAPTER TWELVE

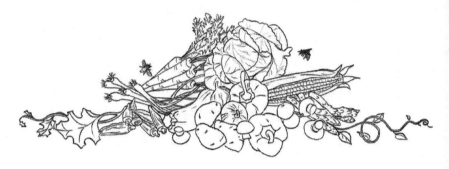

ANTIOXIDANTS

"I used myself as a guinea pig. I saw my energy levels skyrocket, my body fat spiral downward, and my blood pressure and PSA drop like a rock! I fought for my dad's life, I fought for my own, and I'm fighting for yours!"

Antioxidants are the most extremely powerful hidden health treasures on God's green earth. Just as a good fuel injector cleaner cleans out the gummed up fuel lines in our automobiles, natural antioxidants clean out the arteries in our bodies. As I have mentioned many times before, I am not writing this book solely based on the documented research of others, but also on my personal experience of reversing my own health--in a way doctors and modern-day science say is impossible. Antioxidants have played a major role.

I am living the so-called impossible dream, and I want you to live it too. Marketing scams want us to believe that antioxidants are some sort of new invention that we can only get from inflammatory infused drinks, powders, or supplements from a gas station convenience store (poison center). As I mentioned before, I'm not a huge fan of supplements and certainly not fond of any (so-called) nutrient from a fake food producer. We all learned as children how to pronounce almost every natural grown food item on the planet, so why would we be willing to put things in our mouth whose names sound like they came from an industrial supply warehouse? Well guess what--most of them do. And the reason we eat them is called marketing: greed, addiction, politics, and corruption. This is where lobbyists come into the picture. The industrialized food industry spends hundreds of millions of dollars annually lobbying politicians including Congress to allow toxins to be in our food.

Wouldn't it be great if they lobbied for eating more fruits

and vegetables? It's absolutely shameful when a food company engineers something such as a grape flavored sugar water with chemically-made, dangerous liver and thyroid-killing synthetic vitamins, and then calls it an antioxidant drink. Real antioxidant drinks are things like organic unpasteurized fresh-squeezed orange juice, cherry, beet, cranberry, and apple juice, green tea, cinnamon tea, or raw unpasteurized milk--just to name a few of my favorites. When purchasing juice, be sure to examine the label for ingredients. That list should only include the product on the front label. For example, if it calls itself orange juice then it should just list orange juice and only orange juice on the label. It should not even include filtered water because if it does, it is added as a filler to water down your once healthy juice which then is usually labeled as a concentrate blend. CONCENTRATE BLEND=PROFIT!!! NOT GOOD HEALTH.

When purchasing green tea, don't ever choose the ones pre-mixed in a bottle. Yep, those are most likely inflammatory as well. It is safe to say that all tea drinks available at gas stations (poison centers) are inflammatory. Most have hidden sugars, MSG, and or artificial sweeteners and have been processed at high temperatures. Instead of grabbing those, you should shop for whole organic tea leaves, and not the ones in tea bags. A tea bag holding tea leafs (that have been pulverized into powder) leaves more surfaces of the leaf to be exposed to light and air. This allows the polyphenols (antioxidants) to greatly lose their strength, not to mention their natural flavors. Next, never bring your water to a boil for steeping tea. By boiling, you pasteurize the tea which then kills all of the healthy antioxidants that you wanted in the first place. Mass producers of tea suggest on their labels to use boiling water to steep in order to kill bad bacteria in their product. Basically they are suggesting their product is not so healthy and you need to kill it before ingesting it. My answer: just shop for a healthier organic product and never let the water get over 150° for steeping.

Antioxidants come in many forms. You can assume that basically all naturally grown plant foods are considered anti-oxidants. Anytime you consume foods such as organic fruits and vegetables, raw nuts and seeds, wild caught fish, (real) grass-fed meats, raw dairy, and pure unpasteurized juice, then you will have eaten antioxidants. Eating only natural foods eliminates disease causing inflammation, and unwanted body fat immediately starts dissolving out of your body.

On the flipside, if you consume culturally popular foods from mega giant fake food producers and animal feedlots, then you will have eaten herbicides, pesticides, hydrogenated trans fat oils (such as cottonseed), genetically modified corn and soy-beans, pasteurized lifeless dairy, antibiotics, growth hormones, sugar, bleach and preservatives--just to name a few. And your body will be full of disease-causing inflammation.

If you want to know what the difference is between these choices of products and the effects they have on our bodies, refer back to chapter ten and take another look at what the inflammatory salt and foods did to the grass with the inflammatory urine study. Your body reacts no differently than the healthy or dead grass. The state of your health depends on the choices you make for yourself and your family. It's not rocket science and doesn't take multi-million-dollar studies from corrupt mad scientists to tell you how to heal your body.

Antioxidants are all around us, not just limited to whole foods. Something as simple as organic fresh ground peanut butter is loaded with the antioxidant *resveratrol*--the same heart healthy antioxidant that is in purple grapes and wine--but without the alcohol. And don't think for one minute that the inflammatory body-swelling big box store peanut butter is anywhere close to the kind of peanut butter I'm talking about. Most of us who are trying to get healthy and lose weight wouldn't dream of including a peanut butter and jelly sandwich in our diets. I wouldn't either if it came from processed refined fake foods. But my typical peanut butter and jelly sandwich starts with homemade bread, spreading on a generous portion of organic and fresh ground peanut butter and then the jam. Now this is where it starts to get tricky and don't believe for one minute that you can get a healthy jam at your local big-box fake food store. Try this one-minute recipe to make your delicious and healthy jam: put three or four strawberries, a handful of blueberries (or your favorite fruit) and a squirt of local honey in a bowl and mash them with a spoon into what I call the best jam you have ever eaten in your life.

As I have explained over and over again, you can eat the exact same meal from two different sources with vastly different health benefits. One can be from refined foods that will cause your body to gain weight and wreak havoc on your gut bacteria and even lead you to contract serious disease. The same meal from an all-natural source will generate a very productive immune system, keeping you disease-free and very active right through to your very happy and vibrant old age.

I know many of you are convinced that you are gluten-intolerant or are allergic to grains. You may get a stomach ache every time you eat bread and other wheat products and most certainly because your doctor (the guy that's never told you how to eat healthy) has confirmed you are gluten-intolerant. But I have a different and more probable answer for this matter. Nowadays, most food bakeries are using genetically modified grain, which means that the organic nature of the plant has been changed to allow it to be heavily sprayed with bug sprays and weed killers and fertilized with dangerous chemicals, all of which makes it easier for mega food industry giants to mass-produce their crops. (And believe me they are not concerned about what happens to your stomach as a result). Additionally the bread made with this GMO wheat has been gassed with chlorine and washed with bleach (not to mention the other two dozen dangerous inflammatory chemicals added to the baking process). Have you ever just sprayed a little bug killer into your mouth and washed it down with bleach? And regularly I hear folks tell me, "Well John, they wash it after they pick it". (Maybe, but probably not). So you're telling me that you would spray bug spray onto your food, rinse it off a bit and then eat it? Absolutely not. I don't think you would. So why do you eat theirs?

The point I'm trying to make is that these kinds of processed breads will absolutely make anyone's stomach hurt, without a grain allergy or gluten-intolerance. Have you ever thought about what the purpose of bleach is? It kills bacteria. And the kind of bacteria this bleach is killing is not the bad kind--it's killing your good gut bacteria, which in turn will certainly not only give you stomach aches but will actually destroy your whole intestinal tract. Crohn's disease, irritable bowel syndrome, colon cancer, hmmm. Funny how these unhealthy conditions showed up in America quickly after the corruption of our once beautiful wheat fields. Yes, there are a small per-centage of people with celiac and gluten-intolerance, but that number is actually much smaller than doctors diagnose.

Most doctors do not know why your stomach hurts and simply prescribe a prescription drug that negatively affects your body. How many people do you know with irritable bowel syndrome or Crohn's disease who have been cured from a pharmaceutical drug? And just who do you think manufactures the test and associated scores for the test for these diseases. Yep, the same people who keep lowering the accepted levels of cholesterol so everyone in the world is on medication...phar- maceutical companies. Hmmm--do the math folks.

If you really want to know how to heal your intestinal prob- lems, just eat the John Rankin Way! Before you totally quit eating grains and losing the great fiber and insulin metaboliz- ing effect, I beg you to find or make some real bread. The best bread is made with all the parts of the whole grain still attached and with organic wheat that is not genetically modified or sprayed with chemicals. Real bread is baked without vegetable oils, without msg, without sugar and without any other ingre- dient like the words natural flavor or preservatives added. Real healthy bread is made with organic non-gmo wheat, unrefined salt, honey and water--and absolutely nothing else.

Also the myth of the day is that bread (in moderation) will make you fat. Not true! Any real food product (eaten in mod- eration) with as much fiber as this whole wheat grain functions in a manner to only make your body leaner, lower bad cho- lesterol levels, and metabolize your insulin levels. Remember that I'm not talking about the disease-causing bread you have been buying at your local discount grocery store. And as for peanuts--unless you have a peanut allergy, the only concern is that molded nuts can cause some health problems and mold can be found in bad lots of peanuts. This is why I recommend organic fresh ground from a healthy source. And this is true with any food source. You can usually just give the peanuts a quick visual inspection and they will tell the story. Aflatoxin is a carcinogenic mold that is rarely found on peanuts, which is why you want to do a visual inspection. You will probably never see this mold on an organic peanut from a reputable source. Many studies have pointed to the fact that peanut butter is actually a very healthy saturated fat that aids in the cardiovascular system.

One of my favorite antioxidant weapons for energy (endorphins), staying lean, prostate health, and anti-cancer and heart disease is the addition of very hot peppers--capsaicin--to my daily food intake. Most of you are probably gasping at this point and thinking there's just no way you're going to burn your mouth off for a little good nutrition. That's exactly what I said too until I used myself as a guinea pig again. I saw my energy levels skyrocket, body fat spiral downward and my blood pressure and PSA drop like a rock! I won't force you to

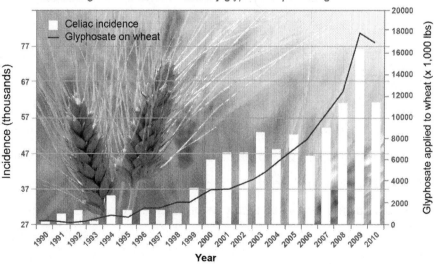

Gluten Intolerance is really GLYPHOSATE POISONING

What if...."gluten intolerance" is really glyphosate poisoning"?

try it, but I highly recommend it.

With the thermogenic effect hot peppers have on our bodies, you could just eat them and sit on the couch all day and still lose more weight than by doing thirty minutes of cardio followed by a fast food meal. Yes, this is great news for all of you spicy food lovers. Hundreds if not thousands of studies have proven that the cayenne pepper (among other varieties) promotes weight loss through a thermogenic effect on your metabolism. This effect is the opposite of what happens to your body when you consume products loaded with caffeine. Caffeine raises your heart rate and blood pressure by restricting the blood vessels and is also extremely dangerous. The products caffeine comes in are usually loaded with hidden processed sugars or artificial sweeteners and dyes that wreak havoc on insulin levels and on your thyroid. Cayenne pepper actually expands your blood vessels while lowering your blood pressure, lowering your heart rate, and kicking up your metabolism levels to full speed at the same time.

Many new studies from Japan, England, and the United States have proven the chemical compound capsaicin (which is in peppers) will prevent and kill prostate, lung and other cancers. Works for me folks! So let me get this straight: I'm a man who can burn my mouth just a little bit by eating a couple of peppers daily and probably never have prostate cancer? (Or I could whine like a baby and cry that it hurts my mouth and risk cancer)! Have you ever considered how much it will hurt if your surgeon has to take a knife to your crotch, slice you open like a piece of sandwich meat (the same meat that caused your cancer), remove your manhood, and inject your body with dangerous chemotherapy and radiation drugs? I have considered this choice, and it didn't take me very long to decide to eat hot capsaicin daily! And that's one of the ways I ended up at sixty years old with a PSA marker of 0.70. One of the things your PSA number represents is the level of inflammation in your prostate gland. Because of my choice to consume peppers daily, my PSA level is equivalent to what a 10-year-old boy would have!

Folks, you have been sold a con that healing is not so simple, but the things I am telling you in this book are the absolute truth. You can have the same blood test results as I have with just a few changes in your diet...or you can just keep taking immune killing antibiotics until you die from prostate cancer. It's really that simple. Take it or leave it.

Pepper also has an anti-platelet-sticking agent in it that helps prevent blood clots from forming in the body. Eat it every day and you can probably throw away the daily aspirin. Smart (honest) scientists are now actually recommending ingesting some cayenne pepper at the onset of a heart attack instead of the aspirin protocol commonly suggested. Scientific studies show pepper is absorbed into the cardiovascular system and opens the arteries much faster through the tiny blood vessels under our tongues and throughout our mouth and esophagus. I can say from personal experience that when I chew on extremely hot peppers, I can actually feel the blood rush in my

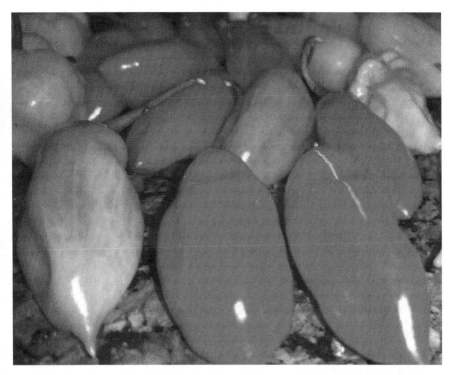

head and watch the arteries on my arms grow larger within one minute. If in doubt, try it and you will see for yourself.

Asian and many other foreign countries eat meals spiced heavily with hot peppers and have much less obesity, heart disease, and cancer--not my theory--just do the math. History and modern-day science prove it. It's also very understandable that some will not or cannot take the burn from capsaicin, and that's why I recommend purchasing cayenne capsules with varying heat units to take with meals. Sometimes I take these when I'm away from home, though I have been spotted many times pulling a bottle of extremely hot pepper powder out of my pocket while working out at the gym! Besides the muscle pumping instant endorphins it gives, it also kills pain and inflammation within minutes. Folks, this pepper remedy may sound a little crazy, but dying young with a senseless man-made disease is crazier. This is especially true when we actually know how to prevent it in the first place!

Another of my favorite antioxidants is organic cacao nibs. A cacao nib is just cocoa before it has been ground into powder from its original pod. Cacao in any form is loaded with extremely healthy plant flavonols which are also found in fruits, vegetables, and also cinnamon, green, and other teas. Many studies show that pure raw cacao has twice the amount of antioxidants as the amount found in a glass of red wine or green tea (so just skip the alcohol). And good news for those of you who struggle with low HDL cholesterol: cocoa has been found to help raise it to a healthy level. Cacao is one of the foods that helped raise my HDL (good cholesterol) from a dangerous low of 29 to a very healthy level of 54 in less than six months time. I recommend adding two tablespoons of cacao nibs into your morning shake or evening yogurt. For those of you who don't enjoy the crunchy nibs, substitute a good organic raw cacao powder. As I have mentioned many times, it is better to get your nutrients whole than from foods that have been pulverized into oblivion. I recommend always choosing foods as close as possible to their natural state, which is more likely to leave all of the healing power of the polyphenols (antioxidants) intact. Never eat store-bought chocolate. I have an excellent homemade chocolate recipe on my website that is very healing, made with all antioxidant ingredients and without any processed sugar. And everyone agrees that they taste wonderful. Carry these delicious natural candies with you daily to help you kick your sugar habit. Consider it your medicine!

What's the first thing you do when you slice open a fresh pineapple or avocado? Well of course you throw away the core and the seed. Pineapple is loaded with rich mineral sources such as vitamin C, manganese and copper, and it also has a naturally occurring protein enzyme called bromelain which has been scientifically proven to reduce inflammation and pain. And it just so happens that the pineapple core has much more of this nutrient than any other part of the fruit. I know that this is not something most folks would want to chew on so here's my idea: cut the core into a half dozen pieces and freeze them, then simply add a piece of the core to be ground with a load of other antioxidant foods in your morning smoothie.

As for the avocado seed that most of us just plunk into the garbage can, save it for your smoothie as well. It has 75% more antioxidant than the fleshy parts. Avocado is a very heart healthy saturated fat and it's a great collagen builder for beautiful skin. Eat them daily if possible. It is loaded with natural fiber, and your intestinal tract, pancreas, and liver will love the natural blood sugar metabolizing effect. I love avocados! I use them as a spread on my hamburgers in place of mayonnaise. The most exciting news about the avocado seed is that according to current studies, it is killing cancer cells in leukemia patients. Imagine that: no immune system killing chemotherapy or radiation, hmm. I'm betting the doctor didn't tell you that one either, if he even knew.

Just remember folks: 100% of the things I speak of in this book will and have been proven to kill cancer, reverse diabetes, and restore heart health--just to mention a few of the extraordinary benefits. That's why God put them here! Please, never be skeptical and wonder if these things are true or not. If you do, then you will fail. You have my sincere word and promise that it worked for me and many others and it will work for you too!

When eating a bell pepper or an orange, most of us usually throw away the stringy white stuff just under the skin. Big mistake. This particular part of the fruit is loaded with minerals, vitamins and phytochemicals. Additionally it is high in flavonoids and super antioxidants that kill free radicals and prevent oxidative damage (disease) to our cells. It really doesn't taste bad either. Try eating all the parts the next time you cut open your fruits and vegetables. Your immune system will love you!

The next antioxidant I highly recommend is cardamom. You would surely think that Americans would have heard about the medicinal properties of something that is considered the queen of spices in India, right? Wrong. Pharmaceutical companies absolutely do not want you to know about the benefits of this product. This small little seed has been known to not only prevent but kill most digestive tract cancers. I personally witnessed these miraculous results with a close friend of mine who was sent home to die with stage four colon cancer before I recommended that she eat cardamom daily. That was four years ago, and she is cured of all cancer and doing well as I write this. Eating cardamom is not an option folks. An added benefit is that it makes your breath smell as fresh as an herb farm.

I would personally rate cardamom as one of the top five anti-oxidants in the world. It was originally grown in India but it is now grown in places like Guatemala as well. It has been used for thousands of years as a natural antibiotic. When you leave a restaurant in those countries, you are offered cardamom for a breath freshener. When you leave a restaurant in the USA, you reach into a bowl and grab a handful of peppermint candy (sugar poisoning) with the excuse that it is for freshening your breath. There's only one problem: as you put the peppermint candy into your mouth, your liver starts swelling like a balloon. Over 37 trillion cells in your body instantly become inflamed, including the cells of your brain, lungs, heart, liver, pancreas and so on. Are you starting to get the picture about processed sugar? As you suck on the peppermint candy, your breath starts to smell great--just when your insulin levels are spiking out of control. After approximately forty-five minutes--about the same time your insulin level crashes--the processed sugar in the mint turns to bad bacteria and your breath smells worse than it would have if you had not eaten it to begin with.

END RESULT? You just caused total inflammation (the cause of 99% of disease) in your body doing something as simple as trying to freshen your breath. Well why not? Haven't we been told (conned) all of our lives that peppermint candy is good for us and freshens our breath? I can only imagine who was behind suggesting such sugar-based remedies. My guess is the mega fake food companies that produce peppermint candy told us through fake so-called scientific studies! Folks please carry some cardamom seeds with you always, and you will reduce your inflammation markers and save your health.

Several recent studies have actually proven that eating cardamom has the potential to prevent and kill colon cancer in its tracks. Studies also show it will heal and prevent most diseases of the intestinal tract, including stomach ulcers, mouth sores and abscessed teeth. Cardamom is also used as a natural flavor enhancer in cooking. In Indian food, cardamom is traditionally mixed with healing ingredients such as raw milk, unrefined salt, turmeric and cayenne pepper and made into tasty sauces. These delicious spicy Indian sauces include many powerful natural anti-inflammatories. In America, the common sauces served include pasteurized (dead) milk, processed sugar, refined sodium, MSG and refined white flour. The proof is in the fact that America's colon cancer rates are as much as eleven times higher than they are in India. Do the math folks. This is not my theory, it's just more truth from history.

Simply chew on a couple of cardamom seeds (inside the pod) after each meal, and if you did happen to encounter a bad bacteria in the meal you just ate, you probably won't even know it. The cardamom will have already killed it. Yes, it's that powerful. Cardamom is also the cat's meow when it

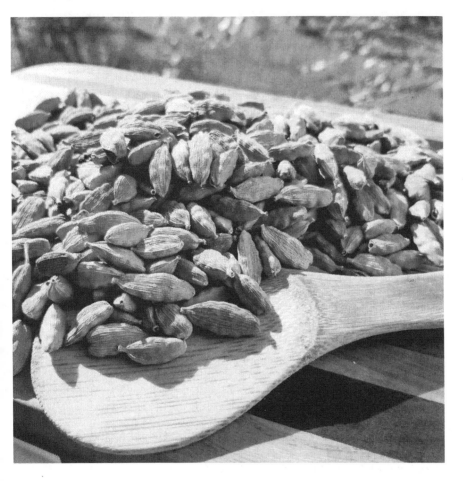

comes to almost instantly stopping acid indigestion, heart-burn and hiccups--and it even helps to lower blood pressure and PSA.

I've spoken a lot already in this book about the natural anti-inflammatory effects of raw unpasteurized dairy, so I will just add here that you're losing the battle big time if you don't check it out.

I never eat white potatoes, sometimes I eat sweet potatoes, but the best potato choice is the Japanese purple yam. Some varieties of these purple skinned and very purple meaty potatoes originated in America, but we don't eat them as a daily staple like the Okinawans, where interestingly, they have more centenarians living than anywhere in the world. The purple yams have approximately 150 times more antioxidants than blueberries and are absolutely loaded with purple phytonutrients. Maybe the nutrients found in purple yams are why those folks live to such a ripe old age? Like I've said before, if someone's doing it better their way, then I just follow them unless and until I come up with something better.

After this next story, I'm going to stop talking about antioxidants for now. I won't give you 300 things you need to take (like every other health-related publication does). That formula is mind-boggling trying to remember everything you're supposed to do, and it just can't work. If it did, you wouldn't be buying this book. I have a different theory that has worked for me and many others. John Rankin's Way is a great guide for anyone (including you) to follow and become very lean and healthy in just a few months!

And now my greatest antioxidant story of them all. At age

thirty-three and only six years after watching my mother slowly die from cancer, my father shocked us by having a horrific stroke. I sadly stood that day and watched my father go from a brilliant beautiful man to a vegetable, in a mere twelve hours in a hospital critical care unit. This is certainly not something I would wish on anyone, but it happened to me and I had to deal with it quickly on that very sad day. It changed me forever.

For the next couple of weeks, doctors told my family and I that my father's chances of living were slim at best. His right side was paralyzed and he could only mumble his words, and naturally no one knew what was going on in his mind. He was eventually sent to a physical therapy center at the hospital, but he wasn't well enough for that. He was getting worse and coughing up most of the fake hospital food they served him. In my repeated vocally expressed concern that it didn't seem like he could swallow his food, the nurses just kept saying he's okay and he will eat his food when he's hungry. Eventually they found out the hard way that I was right and that his swallow muscles were not working in his throat.

But then one night I noticed his catheter was stopped up with what looked like cottage cheese and I kept asking the nurse if that was normal. All these nurses kept insisting he would be okay and not to worry, but it sure looked like a bacterial infection to me. So I temporarily comforted myself by asking, what did I know about this sort of thing at age thirty-three? They are the professionals, right? But remember, it was not my first view of a catheter in a terminally-ill person. I had become well acquainted with the workings of a hospital by this time in my life. I knew something was very wrong.

As the hours passed my father seemed to be getting sicker and the infection seemed to thicken in his catheter, but I was still told over and over by the so-called hospital professionals not to worry, that he would be okay. After some time more, I could just not stand this craziness any longer, so I demanded that a doctor come in and see him late one night. And I was right. When the doctor arrived, my father had a temperature of 104°, his lungs were full of unswallowed food, and a massive bacterial infection had overtaken his body.

Dad was immediately sent to the critical care unit and placed on a special kind of bed that is pumped full of ice water, automatically rolling the patient back and forth. He was pumped full of risky antibiotics intravenously for three straight days until he went into renal failure and his organs started to shut down. He was dying.

The doctor gathered all of my family together and told us that he would not live another day. He said that Dad's organs had shut down and there was no hope for him to live, that we should turn off his ventilator and let him die peacefully. Well at this time in my life I really didn't see anything peaceful about dying, so my brain went into action thinking what to do. I remembered something I had learned from the intensive study I had been doing over the prior thirteen years, inspired by the health issues of my close family members. I had learned that garlic kills bacteria 100% of the time on contact.

My siblings and I could not stand by and let our father die by listening to this doctor's prognosis, giving up and turning off the switch. It's just not in our family's DNA to give up. In our meeting with the doctor, I suggested that we give our father a liquid form of garlic (that one of my sisters just happened to produce and sell). I thought it should be possible to inject it into his feeding tube, so wondering if that would help I asked for permission from the doctor. I told my siblings that we don't have anything to lose, and so after some discussion they went along with my plan. And why wouldn't they? Most folks will try anything to save their parents from certain death!

The doctor reluctantly said it was okay, but it was obvious he was trying his best not to laugh at our plan. In fact I am fairly certain the doc left these grieving middle-aged children thinking, "well there's another one for the books, this family just doesn't understand medicine". What I did understand that sad night was the true fact that modern medicine was not healing my father and that hospital was killing him from poorly attending to his condition. How kind of them to let us try something to save his life since they were the ones letting him die!

I immediately drove straight home, grabbed a bottle of my sister's liquid garlic, and drove straight back to the hospital and immediately poured it into his feeding tube bottle. Even though all bacteria are not the same, I had complete faith, knowing only that garlic kills some bacteria 100% of the time on contact. "This is a good gamble", I thought. Wouldn't you take those odds if it was your family member given up to die?

We sat through that long night waiting and watching for results. Every time the nurse brought a new feeding tube bottle to the room, one of us was there to load it up with heavy amounts of garlic. As the hours passed, we hopefully and impatiently watched the monitors hooked to my father with desperate prayers that this would work. And then within that first twenty-four hours, my father's body seemed to stabilize just enough to keep him barely alive. His organs started to show signs of functioning again. The doctors repeatedly told me not to be hopeful because sometimes this positive turnaround can happen just to see him live only a few days at most. We still watched, prayed, and fed him heavy doses of liquid garlic.

Within seventy-two hours my father's fever had broken and his temperature started downward towards the normal range. His organs started to function even better, and we knew then that the miracle we hoped and prayed for was happening. My father's body started functioning once again as it was meant to do.

The doctor came to our room a few days later and told me that patients can survive this sometimes, almost as if to claim the honor of his healing for himself-- after his insistence to pulling the plug on my father only a few days before. Was it so easy for that doctor to let our beloved father be put to sleep like an injured animal?

This simple little garlic miracle enabled my father to live nine more years of his life. His right side was paralyzed and he was in a wheelchair to get about, but we could converse with him and he seemed happy enough. Would he have been better off dead? God only knows, and it's not up to us to decide. We are put here on earth to give all we have to our life experiences like this one of mine, and to endure well to the end and never give up.

Moral of the story: never be afraid to stand up against adversity. Always do what you know in your heart is best, using the God-given knowledge you have. And don't listen to others who tell you your way won't work when your gut tells you you're right! That's the accountable life, and it's time to take ownership.

Believe me folks, disease should not even be an issue in a country as educated and civilized as America--except for the fact that greedy and conspiring people want to keep doing flawed scientific studies with our funded dollars and not tell us the truth. If they did tell the truth, their job would end. And what do you think is more important: the ending of their job or the ending of your life? I fought for my dad's life, I fought for my own, and I'm fighting for yours!

HEALED BY FARM
CHAPTER THIRTEEN

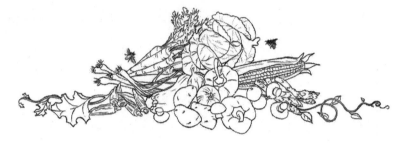

THE BIG CON

"Tombstones don't lie!"

There is one very interesting piece of propaganda that we have been told all of our lives by drug companies, school teachers, and government statistics: because of modern-day medicine, we are living longer today than ever before. We have always thought it to be a fact that prior to the 20th century, humans were smaller than they are now and also were lucky to live much past the age of fifty.

Guess again! This has single-handedly been one of the biggest cons on humanity in the last hundred years. Yes, they got half of it right--humans were smaller a hundred years ago because they hadn't been exposed to a lifetime of growth hormones in every single bite of meat and dairy that they consumed! It is not just a coincidence that humans were mostly smaller before the introduction of growth hormones into our food chain by mega giant dairy, beef, pork, fish and poultry producers. Most of us have probably never given much thought to the fact that we are taller and have much larger feet than our parents and their parents and so on. We have just assumed that we are larger because we are certainly healthier than our ancestors. If this was your belief, you are wrong again, (or technically have been conned once again).

And why in the world would we just assume the potato chip generation that eats the largest percentage of our calories from poison centers (gas stations) would be healthier than generations of the past who consumed 99.9% of their food intake from their own farms and gardens? It's an absolute fact that we are not healthier now. If we were, why do we need to take daily medications for everything from restless inflamed legs to diarrhea? If it were even remotely true that humans suffered as much in past generations as big pharma wants us to believe, humanity would never have had a chance to survive for all these thousands of years.

I can guarantee you that one hundred and fifty years ago, toilet paper stock was not as good an investment as it is today. Television is full of commercials from pharmaceutical companies selling gut destroying medications (that supposedly heal your already destroyed gut). These constant daily advertisements bombard us with their new remedies for everything from irritable bowel syndrome to cramping to constipation. Do you even remotely believe that humans evolved all these thousands of years to have constant diarrhea and cramping?

The good news for all of the folks just like me who eat a 100% clean farm diet: we don't have these modern fake food health issues! Modern pharmaceutical companies are either getting slicker with their advertising or we as consumers are getting dumber--or maybe just conned.

Just to give you a couple of examples of how masterful these pharmaceutical companies are, watch the television advertisement that says this: if your current antidepressant is not working well enough for you, then you can take a second (dangerous medication) that will boost the first one--or the medication that relieves constipation caused by the dangerous pain medication that they already addicted you to in the first place. Come on folks, these companies are masters at selling you the con. Let's stop the madness now.

This is what it's coming down to: pharmaceutical companies earning tens of billions of dollars wasn't enough to cure their greed, so now these same companies are teaching our doctors that they should prescribe you two gut killing drugs per symptom instead of one. I guess their motive is now twice as dangerous as it once was. (In defense of the doctors who I regularly criticize, they only know and do the things they have been taught by big pharma and medical schools-- schools that have been bought and paid for by the mega giant fake food industry).

This is an absolute fact. From coast to coast in America (and other countries where their political lobbying power is beyond control), pharmaceutical and food companies are contributing to the building and teaching staff of medical schools. Doctors are only doing what they have learned in medical school--to prescribe a medication to every patient who comes through the door. This is the same problematic situation of grocery stores selling only what the big manufacturers tell them to sell.

Doctors are not being taught proper or truthful classes on nutrition in school. The only nutrition being taught is a dangerous con from the school's sponsor--and of course that is usually a fake food company. Colleges and medical schools absolutely teach doctors that dead food products are healthy, when most

of the time they are far from it. This is very true when a spon-
sor of big industry is sitting on the board of trustees and also
involved in the educational curriculum. Most Americans are
unaware that this is happening at most American colleges. Just
what do you think happens when a school refuses to teach what
the big mega fake food companies want them to teach? That's
right, the big donations stop immediately. Is this whole picture
starting to look like our big sick nation and the deaths of many
of our loved ones are solely the result of the doings of these
powerful conspiring greedy people? If that is the conclusion
you are coming to then half of my work is done here folks and
we can move along to the healing process much easier.

We have been told since birth from almost all available
sources that the average lifespan of a human was only around
fifty years-old before the 20th century. That is when modern medicine supposedly came to our rescue and saved the
longevity of all mankind. I really try hard not to laugh when
I read these phony twisted statistics, especially when I know
the truth of my own ancestors. My family has been heavily
involved in genealogy for the last three generations, and we
have family records dating back through the past six centuries.
In researching these records, I became aware of several infants
who died at birth and a few middle-aged people who died from
things such as snakebite, lockjaw from stepping on a rusty
nail, or blunt trauma from falling off a horse or wagon. I also
learned from these (uncorrupted) records that a very large

percentage of my ancestors lived to ripe old ages of eighty-five to one-hundred years.

NOW WAIT JUST A MINUTE, CONNED AGAIN? Well that's just what I was thinking, so I took this search another step forward and randomly researched the ages of several famous people who lived pre-20th century. Just imagine what I discovered.

Florence Nightingale (1820-1910).............. lived to be 90

Queen Victoria (1819-1901)......................... lived to be 82

Ralph Waldo Emerson (1803-1882)............. lived to be 79

Harriet Beecher Stowe (1811-1896)............. lived to be 85

John D. Rockefeller (1839-1937)................. lived to be 98

Thomas Edison (1847-1931)........................ lived to be 84

Ben Franklin (1706-1790)............................ lived to be 84

John Adams (1735-1826)............................. lived to be 91

James Madison (1751-1836)........................ lived to be 85

John Quincy Adams (1767-1848)................. lived to be 81

Andrew Jackson (1767-1845)..................... lived to be 78

Some of you may be skeptical of my hypothesis, thinking I just hand-picked the lucky few who lived to be a ripe old age. But to double-check my theory, I decided to go beyond researching the ages of my ancestors and many random famous people. I wanted to go visit some older cemeteries and see what truth lay there for me. These were not just any cemeteries, but some close to my home in a heavenly place called Cades Cove--a pioneer settlement in the Great Smoky Mountains National Park. Well, why not? Folks there lived a very hard life, and did not have access to cities with doctors and medications. They survived living off the land on the naturally available local plant and animal life.

When I began this hunt I was fairly certain that tombstones don't lie, and I was also fairly certain that big pharma had not yet snuck into the cemeteries to change the death dates. So what would you guess that I found? Not surprisingly, most of the people buried there actually lived to ripe old ages (with the exception of a few who had died at childbirth--understandable in those days). What I also discovered was that a European trader by the name of Peter Snyder--one of the first pioneers to settle there--lived to be eighty-seven years old (1776-1863).

So just how in a place so remote and without our modern-day medical help and prescription medicines did Peter live to be eighty-seven years old? I'll tell you how, and it's very simple: he brought along 'ole Bessie the milk cow (leaving the milk unpasteurized of course), chickens, pigs (yes bacon), a backpack full of garden seeds, an axe and a good hunting rifle. And nope, no modern medicine was available or needed for that matter.

Another famous Cades Cove settler was John Oliver. He lived to be seventy (1793-1863) and was a veteran of the war of 1812. Poor old John (who was beat up badly from war) only lived to be seventy years old! And in my personal opinion that is really something to be proud of, especially when big pharma and our government statistics would have us believing that everyone died at forty-five to fifty years of age back in those days. (And as I have mentioned before, surely you are aware of where our government officials get some of their statistics from--yep--big pharmaceutical companies). By the way, John Oliver's wife, Lurena Frazier, lived to be ninety-three years old (1795-1888).

After spending time in the old cemeteries and learning that most of the folks in this area in the nineteenth century had lived to very full and ripe old age, I knew for sure that we had been conned once again. So just how in the world did these poor folks live to be so old without modern-day lifesavers such as pharmaceutical medicine, chlorinated and fluoridated water, and all of the so-called sanitary food processing factories that government statistics say we absolutely cannot live with-out? That's exactly what big industry has convinced us. Our elected leaders and much corruption from big food companies have put almost every healthy small mom-and-pop farm in America out of existence. And just how do you think they accomplished that? Do the math, folks--$$$.

So you might say the handwriting is on the tombstone. You can believe the wealth-hungry pharmaceutical and mega food industry or you can accept the truth. Some folks might just simply say that it is no big deal, that's life, but in my opinion and hopefully yours by now, it is a very big deal! History has been illegally altered just for the financial gain of greedy conspiring con artists who have put you and your loved ones' health at such high risk. These profit-mongering companies have treated us as though we are just another piece of their sick corrupt game--and most of this culture is just standing by ignorantly watching it happen. Age averaging is how the con artist tweaked the numbers to make us believe their lies. In other words, if a hundred people were born in a certain area such as Cades Cove and fifty of them died at birth and the other fifty lived to be a hundred years old, then they announce that the average lifespan in that time was fifty years.

I don't know about you folks (and I'm no great mathematician), but this way of calculating is nothing more than fuzzy math in order to once again trick the consumer into believing something that is totally untrue. So naturally, using that kind of mathematical trickery and the fact that many more babies survive childbirth nowadays, the statistics show (through this false compilation of the data) that humans are living longer.

I do admit the true fact that more babies and mothers are surviving birthing due to doctors and clean and well-equipped birthing rooms, but it is absolutely not due to our modern-day pharmaceuticals. And when you consider the fact that babies are now living longer, the phony averaging of these statistics is being used to show that adults in our day have a higher life expectancy. Please see this as it really is--a CON, CON, CON.

Do the pharmaceutical companies want us to believe that humans have been sick for thousands of years and only now are being saved from death and destruction by consuming their dangerous drugs? This is just simply not true. What they don't tell you is about the tens of thousands of premature deaths of fetuses each year due to the parents consumption of prescription drugs. I'll be willing to bet that you won't see that on any pharmaceutical television commercials anytime soon. All of this phony manipulating of the numbers is just to further the propaganda, and unfortunately we are the ones on the blunt end of this marketing.

Baby boomers were lied to through television food commercials in the 1950's. They started using movie stars and models to make you believe their (poisonous inflammatory) foods would make you look like an athlete--by simply eating a bowl of their (inflammatory) processed cereal. The results of that lifestyle show anything but a healthier generation. Isn't it ironic that sixty years later the advertising of these pharmaceutical commercials make the same baby boomers look enviously healthy, happy, sexy and athletic?

These companies produce endless commercials portraying some guy jumping into a pool or playing ball with the family and looking exceptionally happy, all because their morning pill or insulin shot enabled them to be active and healthy and happy. Don't believe it for one minute, folks. If you are someone who needs to stab a needle into your abdomen twice daily while on a family picnic, you are without a doubt not having fun.

I have spoken with thousands of people about their health problems and the majority of them are not seeing good results. I speak to an exceptionally large number of health-concerned people who have diseases such as hypothyroidism, irritable bowel syndrome, and psoriasis. To some these type of diseases may not seem like such a big deal but believe me they are a big deal and you don't have to suffer with them.

There are pros and cons to these types of diseases. The cons are that if you have been taking prescription medicine prescribed by your doctor for these types of diseases and are seeing no relief, then you have a big problem. NEWSFLASH!! If you are following the so-called modern medical agenda then you absolutely will not see relief, because many of the prescribed drugs actually kill more healthy gut bacteria and compound the problem.

The pros are that if you follow the way that worked for me-- the John Rankin's Way, I can show you how to overcome these problems the natural way without medication. My way actually works, and works very quickly too. What most folks don't understand and doctors usually do not explain is that these so-called small diseases are precursors to something very bad that's about to happen next in your body.

When you have irritable bowel syndrome that lasts for months and even years without relief, you are surely on your way to something much bigger happening in your body than a stomach ache and backed up bowels. Leaky gut is no laughing matter. It seems that half of America has gut issues and just cannot seem to rid themselves of them. The failing of your normally healthy gut means your immune system has crashed to dangerous lows and you are then susceptible to most diseases.

The folks who I speak with tell me their doctor has never mentioned anything worse happening from these bowel syndromes. They just tell their patients to keep drinking the kool-aid. Most of these folks tell me that their doctor just keeps changing the type of gut destroying medication they are taking and hoping that one of them works. It never does--just ask around for yourself.

I guess you have noticed by now that I don't give you the normal look like a fitness model and lose twenty pounds in seven-days diet plan in this book like most self-help books do. I did this for a reason: it doesn't and never has worked for anyone. My John Rankin's Way plan actually does work. I intentionally did not confuse you by telling you every piece of fish, meat, dairy, vegetable, fruit or so-called magical pill to eat like all of the other (health) books. These delicious healing recipes will come later as you follow me.

Calorie-counting and pill-popping absolutely do not heal the human body. We have been told by so-called intelligent scientists and doctors for over sixty years that the only way to lose weight and/or heal your body is to count every calorie that goes into your mouth. This is just totally false. This kind of advice is just another marketing scam to con you to buy so many various so-called health-related fake food products. Give a sigh of relief that you don't ever have to choose from these products or diet again, knowing that god-given real food is easy and simple and the true path to perfect health--not rocket science folks!

Just take a look around when you are in public and see the results of these sixty years of ignorance. LESS THAN EXCITING!! What I share here is simply a logical perspective for how to fix your problems once and for all, healing your immune system (gut bacteria) which in return will heal just about every problem that is anatomically wrong in the human body.

The human immune system is a powerful natural healer that most of us overlook or ignore. Start your way to excellent health by getting your immune system running on over-drive. This is easily done by first eating the proper probiotics naturally abundant in real foods, and secondly ridding your body of processed sugars and inflammatory products. Get as much raw unpasteurized dairy and fermented vegetables (kimchi) as possible into your diet. I can just hear those words of self doubt now, "I don't know where to purchase these items," or "I don't have that kind of time".

Most farm markets in America have the foods you need. If you don't find them then just ask your local farmers. The odds are very good you will succeed. And yes, you will actually have to get your rump out of bed on Saturday morning and make it happen. I can guarantee you it takes less time to shop a farmer's market and prepare and eat their healthy produce than to endure a hospital stay!

I can honestly testify to you that if you keep following the John Rankin Way, you will be pleasantly surprised and you will see results within days--and the rest will come easily. Stay focused folks. Your body is depending on you.

HEALED BY FARM
CHAPTER FOURTEEN

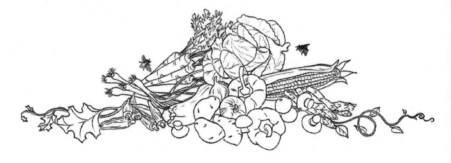

HOW TO FLATLINE FOR TEN SECONDS AND KEEP TALKING

"Advanced stages of any illness does not mean certain death at all."

Modern-day science and most doctors are amazed I did this. It is rather impossible to flatline for ten seconds and keep talking. Those who know me would probably say I do like to talk and could probably do so underwater. I will share the how to shortly, but first let's take a quick look back at my life at that point.

I had been a witness to the deaths of many of my loved ones. First was my grandmother at the hands of my grandfather's stroke which caused that horrific car crash. Then later on, my other grandparents suffered from the effects of diabetes and other inflammatory-causing complications. I had witnessed my mother's long battle and death from cancer, my father's debilitating heart disease and eventual strokes that took him, and next would be the death of my older brother from cancer. I had witnessed my loved ones die from just about every man-made disease that poisonous inflammatory fake food can give us. And because of these experiences, I had made the decision long ago that I would eat healthy and live right on past all of those illnesses. But I also was conned in the fine print. I guess our Creator decided long ago that the ride just wouldn't be nearly as exciting if we were all born with a crystal ball to know all these things from birth. Like all of us, I learned the hard way.

Not long after my fifty-sixth birthday--the years when I was thinking I had been given just about all of the excitement one person can stand in life, I received a call from the ER of a local hospital telling me that my oldest brother was there and that I needed to come and check on him. Within an hour--after a few blood tests and x-rays--the oncologist politely told my other brother and I that he had stage IV cancer with tumors from his brain to his colon.

I vividly remember my brother and I locking eyes like deer in the headlights with knees buckling and tears streaming down our faces. Many of us can relate to this situation and from my past experiences, I was immediately aware what this meant. At that time I was convinced that stage IV anything meant certain death.

Since his death nearly five years ago as of this writing, I have discovered that advanced stages of any illness does not mean certain death at all. It is tragic that any of us have to live through such tragic news being unprepared and uneducated about any means of hope.

My brother was a sugarholic just as I was and just as many if not most of you are now. Neither of us at that time knew or accepted the effects of that addiction. Unfortunately I didn't discover the entire way to heal ourselves from these diseases until after my brother's death, even though I had been trying with every ounce of my ability for over four decades. I had researched the truth about the healing of the human body since I was a very young man, the time when my mother first discovered her cancer and maybe even before. It was also very unfortunate that I had to learn it the good ole-fashioned hard way, almost losing my own life.

When my brother lay in that hospital, I hated to once again listen to doctors tell me face-to-face that there just wasn't anything they could do to save another one of my dying loved ones. I felt so helpless and sick inside. Many of you can relate to this. Looking back I would have been even more enraged and terrified if I had known...my turn was just around the corner.

How sad is it that after decades of so-called cancer research paid for by philanthropists worldwide and all of us participating in thousands of fundraisers like 5k races, all of which have raised billions of dollars--we still don't have a cure!

I hate to say it because it's sickening to think about, but I am starting to believe (fairly certain) this is how it works: researchers get lots of money. If research finds the cure the research funding stops. WAIT JUST A MINUTE, you say no more money? That means no more lifetime job security with perks of mansions, airplanes, yachts and sports cars for the big research companies? Yep that's just what has been happening for a long, long time, with no end in sight. I don't think it makes a lot of sense to keep pouring our money into this kind of researching.

About the time my mother died in 1984, doctors and big pharma researchers assured our family that the cancer that killed her was in the final stages of research and would be cured within no more than five more years. In other words, just keep sending them research money. It was very sad that she couldn't hang on those few more years to be cured by the medical world. Well guess what, conned again. That was over thirty-four years ago and there's still no real true cure for that or most cancers. Do the math folks. As long as the big money keeps flowing in, we will never have cures. Healthy countries around the world (who don't eat fake food) are just shaking their heads at America's health crisis and wondering why we keep running to raise money. They know the cancer cure is just a few steps away in the backyard garden.

Because of my life of family health trials and the resulting deep desire to find the truth about healing, I have without a doubt learned that there actually is a way to save your and your loved ones' lives. And it has absolutely nothing to do with big research money or injecting dangerous inflammatory liver killing chemicals into your veins.

As my brothers coffin was being lowered into the ground, I vividly remember looking at my other brother and two sisters thinking we all looked fairly healthy (especially me!) and that we probably didn't have anything to worry about for a long, long time. What I found out just three months later proved I was somewhat prideful in my evaluation. But it is true that at that time I was a picture of health, having worked out religiously since I was twenty years old and otherwise taken care of myself to the best of my knowledge at the time.

Picture-perfect weight, picture-perfect muscle tone, picture-perfect energy, living the good life....but there was just one problem: I was a certified card-carrying sugarholic. The effects of this addiction were quietly and secretly destroying my healthy body--and that was anything but picture-perfect. I was quickly growing up just like Dad. I had been eating the 'low-fat diet' for some time just like doctors and the American Heart Association recommended, but they hardly ever (or even refused) to discuss or recommend low sugar or no processed foods for good health. I wonder why? Once again...do the math, folks.

Along with my perfect weight, I had a total cholesterol level of 150 and blood pressure of a teenager. Remarkable stats, right? So why would I believe I had anything to worry about? If you had test results like that would you have worried? No, I wasn't worried. Life could not have been better. And right in the midst of all that it's a good life contentment, everything changed. Coasting along one hot summer night in July 2013 and while in the arms of my loving wife, my heart instantly and without warning stopped. Out of nowhere I collapsed unconsciously to the floor. A few minutes later when I became conscious--still lying on the floor--I couldn't understand why I couldn't use my legs or breathe. There is no way to prepare for such a shock.

When something such as this happens without warning, denial comes into play very quickly. I was in denial that I was in trouble, and I had no idea of the horrible mental trauma that my loved ones would suffer. Now I can certainly explain what happens to the human body when the main right coronary artery becomes 100% blocked and you are one hour and ten minutes from arriving at the emergency room. What I can tell you is that when something like this happens to your body, it's game time....and you don't have very long to play.

When I said that my friends would say that I could talk underwater, that wasn't an exaggeration. When a main coronary artery becomes 100% blocked there is no blood going to the lungs...and of course oxygen travels in the blood. Yep--no blood, no air, no breathing, no fun.

Although I had been carted to the hospital more than my share in my lifetime for other things such as bicycle, motorcycle and car wrecks, this time was very different. The difference between this ride and all the others was that I actually thought this was going to be my very last. Does this story sound like fun yet? You better hope and pray it never becomes your story.

For all of you who this may happen to, just be aware that it is just as frightening for your spouse as it is for you. And I was mindful of that as much or more so than my own dangerous situation. So amid my jerking the blood pressure machine off the wall of the ambulance, kicking out of the leg tie-down straps, and screaming at the driver to speed up, I was able to give my wife (who was following in her car) a thumbs up of assurance through the rear glass doors halfway down the road to the hospital.

At that point I was not really sure if I would make it there alive, but felt more emotion for her than myself at that moment. I got the thumbs up idea after following an ambulance that my brother was in from a motorcycle wreck years earlier. Unfortunately, he didn't or couldn't do that little sign for me, so obviously I know that horrific emotion of fear, panic, and trauma of the unknown and worst case possibility very well.

Though a massive heart attack is enough to scare you silly, I think that maybe one of the scariest things when you are rolled into the ER is wondering how much it's going to cost and how you're going to pay for it. (Well, don't worry anymore. That's where I come into your life, teaching you how to prevent disease from ever happening in the first place!) Let's go back to the part in the past chapter when I mentioned how and why tasty, real, healthy food is cheaper than a trip to the hospital. You will know exactly what I'm talking about when you see those six digit hospital bills arrive in your mailbox. Again, it's my sincere passion to keep you from ever getting those hospital bills in the first place.

I have many friends and acquaintances who just simply say, "Well John, I'll just worry about that if and when the time comes." NEWSFLASH!! If you eat only remotely like the rest of the population in our western civilization, your healthcare invoice will be in your mailbox soon. That's not a threat or my opinion--it's a fact. Most of the folks who think this way are the same ones who often excuse themselves by saying, "You have to die sometime". That's very true. But on the other hand, how and what you eat determines how you take care of your health and how much you love your family. They are the ones who will be left with a couple of hundred thousand dollars worth of hospital bills as you lay dying from a senseless disease that you could've prevented in the first place. Or even worse, that your spouse has to push you around in a wheelchair for several years while you are brain-dead, simply because you intentionally and irresponsibly neglected your health!

Besides the fact that I love my wife and children dearly and wasn't ready to depart from this world, I thought about all of these things as I lay in the ER and heard the "beep, beep, beep" on the ECG heart monitor machine turn into a "BEEEEEEEEEEEP." Of course at first I was just thinking that one of my wires had come loose, only to frantically learn really quickly that it was game time once again as the oxygen quickly left my lungs. Interesting how that makes me now appreciate every breath I take.

If you are in denial that something like this will ever happen to you and that you will ever see those medical bills on your kitchen table, think again. I was in denial also, until my eyes were locked onto my dear wife's eyes while four nurses and an ER doctor frantically started my heart that had completely stopped for the past ten seconds--while some guy stood there at the end of my bed with the electrode paddles just itching to shock me. I had seen this happen many times on medical television shows, and I just wasn't about to let it happen to me.

It's amazing how many prayers you can say in ten seconds.

The doctor and staff told me afterwards that a miracle had happened, and they wanted to know just how I stayed conscious and talking (screaming) during that traumatic time. While the average human body becomes unconscious after about three seconds of no heartbeat, I had talked and remained conscious for ten (not exactly the most enjoyable ten seconds of my life). This is where the exercise comes in. I told him that I didn't want to die and leave my wife and children and certainly did not want to get shocked silly by that scary defibrillator guy. And besides that, it was probably because I had been an avid fan of hard workouts at the gym for the past three and a half decades. I was in great shape, so that's why I could still talk. Since this was only the second time he had seen this happen in his thirty-two-year career, he wasn't buying that answer. I admitted that I was fairly certain there was also some divine intervention, to which he smiled and agreed.

After many years of study and observation and good habits, I was as confused as anyone as to why it was me lying there in that condition instead of some sick old fat guy. And after a four-day hospital stay in a bed that was six inches shorter than me--with hoses, tubes, needles and ugly scary things attached to all parts of my body--I came to the conclusion that I would never put my loved ones or myself through this again. I was certainly going to get to the bottom of this.

In the coming weeks, months, and years afterwards, I

poured myself into research to learn more. This research consumed every waking moment, as I looked for the answers no
one could give me (not even doctors). I knew there was a way
to be well and to live without disease. I knew God didn't send
us to this earth to suffer so much illness. I knew it shouldn't be
this complicated. And it isn't. Like the IRS tax code, healthcare in America these days is extremely over-complicated (for
profitable marketing), but I learned the truth--and the truth is
very simple.

I experimented on myself month after month. I wanted
my blood markers to improve, even though American medical
science and doctors said it couldn't be done. (That's something
you never say to John Rankin, by the way.)

As I continued my intense researching, it soon became very
obvious that my situation was 100% caused by the continuous
poisoning of my body from eating (so-called) foods from the
conspiring crooked mega-giant fake food industry. I then took
a quote from the 1976 drama film 'Network'--the part when
people opened their windows and screamed, "I'M MAD AS
HELL AND I'M NOT GOING TO TAKE THIS ANYMORE".

Trust me folks--I'm mad and you should be too. I'm mad
enough that I made the decision to heal my body with only
healing whole foods, without dangerous gut-killing prescription drugs. I'm also mad enough to warn you to beware of the
conspiring ways our politicians, doctors, food and pharmaceutical companies are allowing chemical, unhealthy so-called

food products into our economy for incredible profit. Unaware, our neighbors and loved-ones are becoming unnecessarily very, very, sick, and worse. I am also mad enough that I decided to take my passion one step farther and give freely of my time and experience to educate and teach as many good truth-seeking people as possible. I am now working full-time passionately teaching everyone interested about the horrific hidden dangers that have crept into our lives like enemies in the night.

Surely by now, some of you are wondering why is it that if I have studied these things for over four decades, why could I not have learned these things before and prevented this from happening to myself? Here's the simple easy answer: as healthy as I was and as careful as I was to eat what I thought was healthy, I was still addicted to processed sugars and foods with hidden sugars and chemicals, just like you are. I also had the attitude--just like you have--that since I was physically fit and felt great, it would never happen to me.

The people who are close to me in my life have come to re-alize that this lifelong passion and venture of mine has become an extreme reality. I sincerely hope and pray that those closest to me also realize how much I love and care for them and will do anything in my power to prevent something tragic like this from happening to them. I also hope and pray that you realize I have walked the walk and have actually cured disease with my new way. I have always enjoyed life and considered myself to be a good person, but I spent the first two-thirds of my life making myself the center of attention in my world. Now I have decided that if I cannot spend the last third of my life helping others with this wonderful gift, then I have failed.

In order to learn what is true, I have spent the last four plus years as my own human guinea pig, by choice experimenting with possibilities for healing my body. I have learned that fake food companies, doctors, paid-for scientists, pharmaceutical companies and some of our government officials have been hiding the truth for profit. I would like to thank my family, friends, and acquaintances for trusting me by also being my personal guinea pigs. Many close to me have put their own health in my hands by taking my advice, not to mention all of the hours they have patiently listened to and considered my findings, my stories, and my words of wisdom.

Remember, blood tests don't lie. As you change your eating habits you will most definitely see your blood test numbers change for the better. Your life will return to an energetic and healthy normal. For those of you who have not yet taken my advice, please be aware that I care deeply about you and your health. I advise you to get regular blood tests to see for yourself how changing your diet makes all the difference. Use your blood results as a personal challenge. I hope you will always be on the lookout for all the ways conspiring mega giant fake food companies market you with their propaganda. False marketing and political payoffs have most likely ruined the health and taken the lives of millions of people eating those poisonous inflammatory fake so-called foods.

In your search for good health, I advise you to constantly search out healthy foods, to frequently visit your farmer's markets, grow your own gardens, and to lobby your politicians to get off the backs of small mom-and-pop healthy farmers that nourish and heal our families. I also advise you to get more blood tests than your annual physical and to weigh yourself daily. One very important thing to remember is that real farm-raised food saved my life, and real farm-raised food will save yours too.

HEALED BY FARM
EPILOGUE

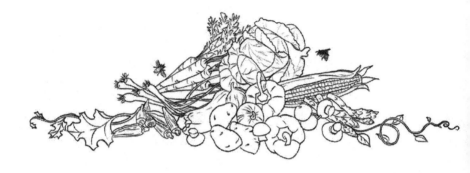

GET HEALTHY AMERICA!

"We are watching our helpless innocent children become obese diabetics. We are watching our parents die too soon from senseless and previously unheard of and horrific diseases. And we are walking in a field of landmines ourselves."

It is now time for you to step up to the plate America. Do you think your healthcare expenses are out of control now? Just wait until the baby boomers retire....the millions of Americans who have been poisoning their bodies from addictions to fake and fast foods for the past six decades!

Do you remember when I said it's game time and not long to play? Well guess what...that time is now folks. We get healthy by educating ourselves and getting involved, refusing to eat the junk food that is so heavily marketed to us. Our so-called trusted media isn't ever going to tell you the truth. And why would they? Guess who signs their paychecks?

For the last time I'm asking you to do the math folks. That's right, how many fast food and pharmaceutical commercials do you watch daily? It's extremely sad that because of the abusive power of the manufacturing, marketing, and lobbying food in-dustry, we are watching our helpless innocent children become obese diabetics. We are watching our parents die too soon from senseless and previously unheard of and horrific diseases. And we are walking in a field of landmines ourselves.

I need your support folks. Follow me and I will stand up and fight for your God-given right to eat clean healthy wholesome food and to never be sick again. After reading this book I hope you will make a personal choice to eat clean and that you will join me in saying:

"Yes we are so done with being lied to and used as guinea pigs by these conspiring companies. We are so done with the abuse of being addicted to fake food. We are not going to let the food (chemical) companies conspire to turn us into can-cered-up diabetics and overweight heart patients anymore. We will choose only pure whole foods for ourselves and our fami-lies. We choose excellent health over addiction."

Thank you for reading and allowing me to share my story and my lifelong experience with you. I hope you will join me in following the John Rankin's Way Back, which is really only a return to eating the way our ancestors did--the way our Creator intended when designing our lives on this earth from the beginning!

I sincerely hope and pray that the moments of pain I suf-fered for my wake-up call--and the lessons learned since--will inspire you and your family to enjoy a lifetime of gloriously good health for yourselves. God bless and .....

GET HEALTHY, AMERICA!

THE AUTHOR'S STORY

JOHN RANKIN'S WAY

John Rankin's Way was created when John totally reversed heart disease after a near-death experience. He tells how he not only shocked his doctors from his initial survival, but how he dramatically changed his blood tests in less than a year from heart-attack levels to those of a healthy child's. His success is credited to his doing the exact opposite of what the medical associations suggest that patients do in cases like his. He began eating like his ancestors did in the 1700's (the John Rankin Way) because–unlike what modern history reports– except for infant and early childhood mortalities, folks in that day actually lived into their 90's. Because of his discoveries, he even ate foods that medical associations had been warning for over 75 years would cause heart disease. Nine months after the "attack," John was preparing to take himself off the required heart-stint life-time-maintenance medications that his doctor and the medication association suggest as the only way to stay alive, when his doctor was so impressed with his healing prog- ress and his lab test results, he took John off all prescription medicines himself. While most medical professionals are in amazement at this reality and say this is nearly impossible, John continues to thrive and shine in perfect health--and need- less to say is the new poster child for that cardiologist!

At the time of his heart attack, John had been studying and following the wisdom of the best in diet and nutrition for over 40 years, except for a few surprising things which he now understands as vital to life, including but not limited to: 1) he had stopped eating healthy saturated fats at the advice of doctors, heart associations and cancer associations and, 2) he was an obvious sugar-holic (just like most Americans and now like most of the world). He had been a regular fitness-junkie, working out 5 days a week and was very active in outdoor adventures of every kind: water and snow skiing, biking, hiking, on and off-road cycling, hunting and just about anything offered to challenge his fitness prowess. In light of having lived such a healthy lifestyle for all those years, then having the 'attack,' John set out to discover how such a life-threatening event could have happened to someone like him. And that's what awakened him to his current life purpose.

John is a self-made man, very gifted and successful in developing his own businesses over the years, allowing his family to live a comfortable life on a lovely wooded property which friends and family have fondly named "Rankinshire." The dream continues there as he practices what he preaches, now raising as much of his own food sources as possible and buying the rest from local approved farmers. The beautiful hills and valleys of East Tennessee have been home to his ancestral family since the 1700's when the Rankin clan emigrated from Scotland and Ireland, and he is proud to continue their traditions of living off the land in a healthy lifestyle.

After John witnessed the death of his parents, brother, and other close relatives from diseases which he believes were caused by the industrialization of the American food industry, and after his own shocking attack as well, he has now chosen to put his full time and attention into this endeavor as his greatest passion. He is committed full-time to sharing the God-given truth about food to all who desire to improve their health, teaching so everyone can have access to vital and yet simple ways of food wisdom. He sets himself up as proof that these truths work, as his body fat reduced from 18.5 to 11% and his perfect lab tests continue to show. You can't help but believe he definitely has something you need to know as you listen to him teach and feel his passion for these truths and his concern for every human being.

John is passionately engaged in a very active speaking tour and creating seminars to teach the details of the John Rankin Way. He is being recorded regularly, with podcasts, articles, and recipes prepared that explain his WAY, which you can continue to access on his website (JohnRankinsWayBack.com).

John calls his many followers 'converts,' because they too have changed their eating habits and healed their own illnesses including irritable bowel syndrome, arthritis, prostate disease, cancer, blood pressure, diabetes, depression, and more. People who listen to and follow "John Rankin's Way" say he is extremely inspiring and knowledgable, as well as individually and personally caring about them. They say finding John is the most wonderful thing that has happened to them, that after listening to him they can't help but act on the wisdom. Even nay-sayers soften and humble, shifting into making better choices after listening to even an hour of his passionate presentation.

Want to lose weight? Want your brain to become clear again? Want to stop worrying about getting illnesses and diseases? Want to stop taking prescription drugs? Want to have unstoppable energy supplies and feel like a kid again? Enjoy this book and stay tuned for more!

Made in the USA
Lexington, KY
26 February 2019